ENJOY

A New Approach To Stress
And Burnout Prevention

ENJOY

A New Approach To Stress
And Burnout Prevention

A strength-based process that
celebrates our uniqueness

Nicole M. Seichter

Niche Presswors

For permission to reprint portions of this content or bulk purchases, contact Nicole M. Seichter at nicole@strengths4you.com

Published by Niche Pressworks; http://NichePressworks.com

ISBN Print: 978-1-946533-13-5
ISBN Digital: 978-1-946533-14-2

Dedication

Daddy—I love you so much! Thank you for everything!

"Do what you can do—today!

Change what you can change—today!

You never know what tomorrow will bring!"

(Nicole M. Seichter)

Contents

Contents

Foreword

Nicole Seichter is a dedicated, passionate Gallup-Certified Strengths Coach, who has a wealth of knowledge and experience helping individuals manage and alleviate stress and burnout in their work and personal lives. I met Nicole during a Gallup Accelerated Strengths Coaching course in Chicago in 2015. Little did we know that this phenomenal course would give us a new and unique perspective of how we view others, as well as ourselves. I can remember Nicole during this course, always asking thought provoking questions about the possibility and value of a person understanding one's talent and leveraging their talents to manage stress and burnout in their lives.

We have all at one time or another experienced stress and/or burnout. Maybe you are experiencing stress or burnout right now. You are about to read a great book with a unique approach to managing stress and burnout like no other book on this subject matter. Nicole has found the value of embracing our uniqueness and has tapped into a unique methodology to help individuals develop a stress and burnout prevention plan using the ENJOY acronym (Embrace, Nurture, Jump, Organize, and You). This book is a must read for anyone seeking to manage stress and burnout in their lives, and for those who mentor or coach someone attempting to manage stress and burnout. Thank you, Nicole Seichter, for this honor and opportunity to write the foreword for your wonderful book, *Enjoy*!

    - BEVERLY GRIFFETH-BRYANT, Gallup-Certified Strengths Coach.

My Equation for Hope

Human Uniqueness = Stress Prevention

Has someone already shared this idea with you? Let me clarify what I mean:

The more you know about yourself and the power of your own uniqueness, the more you are prepared to face the stress and challenges of life. And by this, prevent and protect yourself from stress and burnout.

I am convinced that each person's uniqueness holds the key to their burning desire and capabilities to ENJOY life to the fullest. It is this your own human uniqueness that contains the unbeatable power to conquer any challenge and any stress that may come your way.

This book is my baby; my story. Within its pages, you will read about the ENJOY process which will help you learn to use your uniqueness as an advantage, instead of ignoring it or worse, abusing yourself or others with your behavior. At this point, I want to share with you the big why, there are 2 reasons why I've put this together for you!

Reason Number One:

I am a very empathetic person. In the language of Clifton Strengths®, which I will explain later, my #1 talent theme is Empathy®. This talent helps you read the emotions of the people around you like a book. Words are not needed to know what is happening around you and I'm not shy talking about what I am feeling. It's a great talent, but it can make others feel uncomfortable if they can't, or don't embrace what it can mean for them or their team.

Until I was "introduced" to Clifton Strengths®, I felt wrong so many times. Even being a very positive person with a great amount of energy, my uniqueness was too much for many of the people around me to handle. Early in my childhood, my grandmother used to say to my parents, "She is something … you will be surprised about her." But unfortunately, she didn't mean it in a positive way. I was never normal. This was not accepted, and it has caused me a great deal of stress over the years.

People are easier to deal with if they are adjusting themselves to others instead of staying strong and courageously walking their own path. That being said, I lost a couple of so-called "friends" along my path. Painful. I thought it was my fault, that I did something wrong. But the reason was so simple: I was staying strong and confident in what God created within me. And, I know I'm not the only one feeling this way. This book should be a crutch for you to continue your path, instead of trying to live the life of someone else on this planet.

Reason Number Two:

Every person—every human being has their own story to tell; their own uniqueness, their own perfections and imperfections. The way people ignored my uniqueness—intentional or unintentional—was very painful for me. But what left me speechless over the years, was the fact that others experienced the same issue, but didn't have the courage to stand up for themselves. My #2 Clifton Strengths® is Connectedness®. The power of this talent theme is the capability to discover the bigger picture—to see connections between actions, reactions, behaviors, people, and events that most people don't notice.

Instead of focusing on their own development, some people prefer to accept the fact that they must obey and do what others expect them to do to "get ahead" in life. They cannot use their own uniqueness. That makes them feel weak, wrong, and bad. But since they cannot deal with these feelings, they tend to take their frustrations out on others. Stepping on the backs of others and treating them in the same way they have been treated becomes common practice—a vicious cycle of negative behavior. They fall into their fight or flight mode—get stressed and limit their own options to find the best way to deal with their challenges. And the spiral continues to turn ... I can feel their pain and how their behavior created an environment of stress and negativity—and eventually burnout.

Step by step, I started to come up with the idea that this so-called "weakness" could be the most powerful stress prevention technique ever. There is a reason why you are different. So, how could I help people smile more? This was the initial reason for my decision to become a coach. I wanted to help people to have a real smile on their faces. A smile from deep inside, because they truly FEEL happy. I knew in my heart that if everyone knew that it is ok to be different, and if there was a way to do this on a daily basis, happiness could become a permanent feature in everyone's lives. It would give you the courage to be nice but bold.

If we all knew the definition of our own uniqueness, we wouldn't feel the need to step on others, to BE bigger or more important or to win every argument. Their own unique characteristics would be the self-charging battery for everyone—to create teams on a different level—with a different level of appreciation and recognition.

I was positive this would change the communication in our daily lives. But most importantly, in the workplace. And with less pressure and stress at work, people could continue to develop their personal lives and careers. There would not be the need for a fight or flight reaction as you have been used to. Not creating stress in the first place is the most effective stress prevention of all.

I collected a lot of tools during my career as a coach. I was successful but was still missing the language to explain my theory. The moment I learned about Clifton Strengths®, I knew I had found what I was looking for. Finally, everyone could understand AND explain what is needed to be truly happy—to have a smile on their face. From deep inside, by being yourself!

Uniqueness = Happiness = Stress Prevention

This is Why I Created ENJOY!

E - Embrace who you are

N - Nurture your uniqueness to create your own stress prevention shields

J - Jump and design YOUR plan to BE your true self

O - Optimize your life according to who you are

Y - You, because it all begins and ends with you

Uniqueness = Happiness = Stress Prevention = ENJOY

What is Different About ENJOY?

At Home

You will finally understand what is special and unique about you. Finally, you will get a better understanding of what makes you special. It will help you to explain your uniqueness to others, and express what you need and want to be your best self. And—even better—ENJOY is a guide for you to create a personal development plan. A plan you can work with.

This plan will change the way you feel about yourself, the way you communicate with your loved ones and will improve your efficiency to get things done. This process will change the way you are present in the here and now. This will be YOUR key to live life to the fullest.

At Work

Having this plan and knowing your own uniqueness will help you see that there is beauty and uniqueness in everyone. As an individual—as well as a manager and a colleague. It will change the way you express your needs to others and understand and accept the needs of others.

Knowing about this will support you as a manager and help you to provide your coworkers with the opportunity to do what they do best every day. It's your responsibility to care for your employees. ENJOY is the unique process to help you with this! With ENJOY, every employee will know their own talents and can develop a unique plan to transform the talents into strengths; at the same time everyone can develop a plan for the personal improvement.

The ENJOY process is a tool that will bring joy, laughter and appreciation back into your work environment. These are the conditions necessary to have successful results at the end of the year—and isn't this what you are really accountable for? ENJOY will support you in your work—simple as that—helping you to be more efficient, engaging and pleasing for everyone!

But ENJOY goes way beyond this! Applying the knowledge, you will gain while going through the ENJOY process will boost stress and burnout prevention to a completely new level. It will inspire you to use your individual uniqueness to understand what may create stress and even more importantly, how to avoid it.

It supports everyone in creating their own stress protection shields and therefore brings a powerful self-awareness for everyone involved in the ENJOY process. The ENJOY process will be your assistant to design your personal plan which prepares you not just for stress—but for a self-paced life.

You are part of something bigger—you are part of the system. And, if you change your system, and others change their systems, eventually you will change the whole system, one person at a time!

ENJOY comes with the message: celebrating human uniqueness prepares you for the challenges of your future! That is my equation for hope!

A short note at this point. This book is my creation. It was written with all of my senses and talents. And, of course, it was also written using the lenses through which I see the world. All notes as well as all actions have therefore been written from a perspective of Empathy®, Connectedness®, Maximizer®, Learner®, Positivity®, Adaptability®,

Developer®, Activator®, Belief®, and Woo®, all of which are my dominant themes.

Thank you for reading my book, I really appreciate the time you are investing in learning about the ENJOY process! I invite you to read it from cover to cover, or pick just a few chapters that interest you the most. You have the choice. As you are unique, you will have your own way of doing it! ENJOY! Let's get started! You can do it!

CHAPTER 1

Let's Connect the Dots

My Theory: We Can't go on Like This

Several worldwide health reports[1] confirm the fact that the follow-up costs of long-term illnesses are increasing. The actions and approaches taken to reduce the costs—or to eliminate the causes of these costs—obviously do not influence what is happening. People experience more and more stress and burnout every day.

A system, according to Wikipedia is "a set of interacting or interdependent component parts forming a complex whole." In this case, the set of interacting components is people and the tools they need to secure their health on this planet. That is what I refer to when using the term "system."

Is it possible that the system was achieving or changing something up until now? I would say no. This is why it is necessary to reevaluate the system. As Einstein said, "We cannot solve our problems with the same

---

[1]   Techniker Krankenkasse, Germany, World Health Organization

thinking we used when we created them". We have to change the level; take a step back and link preexisting facts with each other in a new way. It can't go on like this.

If you are blaming everyone and everything else for your own situation, I would venture to say you should turn around and face the facts. The only person responsible for your stress and burnout is YOU. It's not your job, it's not your spouse, it's not the financial situation, or your kids. The workplace and your relationships with others are simply where the problem becomes apparent.

It's not about others – it's all about you.

My Idea: Understand Your Zones!

Most previous approaches for stress and burnout prevention are based on the idea that people should compensate for their weaknesses, find out what did not work, and use relaxation techniques to find the strength necessary to face their challenges. What is missing entirely in this equation is individuality and uniqueness.

There is only one way to get a grip on stress and burnout in the long run—you have to give the human element the value it deserves. You must acknowledge that you are not a carbon copy of someone else. You have unique strengths and weaknesses. YOU ARE UNIQUE!

As we move forward, you will be confronted with the terms "talent" and "strength". You will get an extended explanation of each of these terms and the difference between them in Chapter 2: ENJOY - Step by Step.

At this point it's enough to know that a talent is something you are born with. It can be developed and become a real strength for you if you are aware of this talent, embrace it, and know the steps needed to develop this natural talent into a present and supportive strength. The definition of a strength[2] is: *the ability to consistently produce a positive outcome.* A talent[3] is naturally in you – *a naturally recurring pattern of thought, feeling and behavior that can be productively applied -* whereas, a strength is something you are aware of and know how to use to your advantage.

In his book, *Soar with Your Strengths*, Donald O. Clifton writes, "Burnout is often the mental and physical result of working in an area of weakness; it is final proof that a weakness exists. Burnout is produced by the resistance you experience when you are doing what you're not good at."[4]

When you focus in the areas of your strengths, you have a better chance of staying healthy. If you can recognize your talents, and use them, you will be fulfilled. Understanding each of your talents and what makes them successful, you can use this insight as a key to open the treasure chest of your life.

The more you use a natural and innate talent you are born with, the less energy you have to exert to reach your goals. If it is natural, it requires almost no effort—and gives you joy and energy—to do even more of what you are already doing.

Due to your talents and skills, you have a comfort zone that is totally unique to you. Your comfort zone is that place where you feel safe or at ease without stress, and are in complete control. Here, you have the

---

[2]   Rath, T. (2007). StrengthsFinder 2.0. New York: Gallup Press.

[3]   Rath, T. (2007). StrengthsFinder 2.0. New York: Gallup Press.

[4]   Clifton, D. O., & Nelson, P. (1992). *Soar with your strengths.* New York, N.Y.: Delacorte Press.

opportunity to recover emotionally and to gain the energy you need to face upcoming challenges. However, you may not know your comfort zone very well. Until today, no one could explain exactly where it is, how to get there, or how best to use it. But it is crucial; your comfort zone defines you!

The exact opposite is true of your panic zone. Your panic zone is a place where you feel stressed, tense, and fearful. Panic equals stress for your emotional brain. From an emotional standpoint, it is only about survival. Here, you are helpless and powerless to act with creativity and purpose. The only thing you can do is react. This is not a good place to make decisions, you do not have enough flexibility to do so.

In between these two zones is the learning zone, also referred to as the stretching/learning zone. In this zone, you are challenged to learn and grow, you have your best skills available to you in this zone. Neither boredom nor panic are prevalent here. This is where development takes place; where personal growth happens. You can act and react with creativity and courage. Your brain can access all kinds of information it has gathered over the years.

Your goal should be to avoid the panic zone—instead, you should try to stay in either the comfort or the learning zone, and switch between the two.

When you are working in these zones, you have a solid and stable foundation to live your life and to complete what you need, and are able to do. This increases your self-assurance and minimizes the risk of having to experience stress. You live your life.

If you don't work in your comfort zone, this can lead to stress and even worse, to burnout!

You have a lot of reasons for questioning the old system and for redefining it. The most important reason is YOU. You owe this to yourself. After all, you only have this one life to live. Every second of it is worth asking again and again, "What can I do to become a better version of myself and be able to live the best possible life?"

You are not at the mercy of stress. This is the message of this book— in addition to providing instructions for what each and every one of us can do.

The ENJOY process creates awareness and makes it possible, with the help of your natural talents, to get to know and explore your own learning zone in order to expand it as much as possible. It helps you to experience more personal growth. With the ENJOY process you will create your personal development plan.

CHAPTER 2

ENJOY—Step by Step

Positive Psychology

The ENJOY process is based on positive psychology because this is who I am. One of my dominant Clifton Strengths® talent themes is Positivity®. People with strong Positivity® talents are generous with smiles and are always on the lookout for the upside of any situation. It is why I am who I am, always looking for something positive in every situation and each individual without having read books about it. It is how I naturally approach people and situations.

Unconsciously and intuitively, I pursued and promoted the line of thought mentioned for the first time by Abraham Maslow.[5] In 1954, he introduced so-called "positive psychology."

In contrast to traditional deficit-oriented psychology, which constantly looks for what is missing, positive psychology focuses on what strengths you have and what things you are good at. I was convinced

---

[5] Maslow, A. H. (1970). Motivation and personality. New York: Harper & Row.

that this was the path you have to take to change the system. I just didn't know how to phrase what seemed so clear to me—I was missing the language for it!

Positive psychology motivates us to see the beauty in things and how to get more of it—because this is the path towards real success. It looks at the areas in which you are successful and how and what you can do to repeat success.

It simply matches what I believe in: that there is so much more possible, if you can focus on what is good instead of complaining about what is not working. The reason is simple, it has been proven that people in a good mood are much more creative because there are no limits or boundaries to finding the needed information in your brain. A negative mood creates stress and activates the sympathetic nervous system, which results in a limited ability to find solutions for problems.

This is exactly where Don Clifton's line of thinking and his statement, "What will happen when we think about what is right with people rather than fixating on what is wrong with them?" comes in. Based on Don Clifton's insights, Gallup intentionally researched human strengths and success for 5 decades and recorded the insights they gained. Gallup was the first company that wrote the "Book of Strengths"—literally. The Clifton Strengths® 2.0!

From birth, there are different combinations of talent themes that are responsible for how you think, act, and feel. You are a unique mosaic—that is a fact; and it should be acknowledged and appreciated. Each and every one of our steps and actions is determined by our unique combination of talents and skills!

The day I learned about Clifton Strengths® was almost the best day of my life. I found the language I needed to explain to everyone how every human being is unique. It became the foundation of my work!

Clifton Strengths® is the language to explain human uniqueness, while ENJOY is the process using Clifton Strengths® for stress and burnout prevention. You are much more likely to feel that you have a great life and are far more effective in what you do, if you are who you are and can use the tools you have been given by God.

Maybe this helps: if you are used to eating with a fork and knife, and suddenly you are given chopsticks for the first time, you would certainly struggle to eat! You would be frustrated and that would raise your stress level.

If you know and can explain what makes you unique, your comfort zone is solid and strong to protect you from stress. You must be motivated by the question, "How do I become a better version of myself?"—and not by the question, "How can I become as good or better than someone else?"

The Essence of ENJOY

Every individual has the opportunity to get to know and to understand himself or herself and use this to prevent stress.

- Knowing your talents and how they prevent you from feeling stressed, gives you the opportunity to explain to other people why you act or feel a certain way. This provides you with self-confidence and gives you hope.

- ENJOY is a brilliant and unique way to improve personal performance and create YOUR own powerful comfort zone. It is liberating to know how to explain your unique self; it opens up new opportunities and you become a freer you. Stress is often only caused when you try to be or become someone you admire—someone other than yourself. Or, if you try at all costs to achieve something that does not suit you.

- ENJOY is a simple process that includes the individual beautiful facets of your personality. Enjoy takes your needs into account to create a personal plan tailored for you to prevent stress.

- ENJOY helps us maximize the potential in each individual and the individual takes center stage—this is a huge advantage in the workplace—each individual will multiply their efforts for the sake of the organization.

- ENJOY helps you to gain full control over your own life, and to develop greater awareness of yourself, your feelings, and your behavior. With the right stress and burnout prevention tools, at the right time, you have a solid foundation you KNOW you can count on.

- ENJOY paves the way for strong independence—for people and their lives—and supports your desire to ENJOY life to the fullest. In my opinion, it is the **only** promising way for effective stress and burnout prevention.

- ENJOY will allow employers to offer Clifton Strengths® and effective stress prevention to its employees—just by creating a personal development plan with them. What a great way to care for the most important asset an organization has.

What You Need to Know:

- Clifton Strengths® gives you the framework for developing innate talents into real strengths. It allows you to show your uniqueness in an impressive way. You can find the online Clifton Strengths® assessment at www.gallupstrengthscenter.com. You can also find the link on my homepage at www.strengths4you.com.

- After you have answered all 177 pairs of statements, you will receive different reports. They are the greatest tools to help start your personal development: the beginning. They will help you recognize what exactly is special about you and your talents. However, these reports are only the start of your personal development.

What is the Difference Between a Talent and a Strength?

TALENT	STRENGTH
"A talent is a natural way of thinking, feeling, and behaving."[6]	A strength is the "ability to consistently provide near-perfect performance".[7]
It is about the individual, what makes us unique?	It is about the execution—about HOW we are using the talents.
Who are you?	How do you do it?
Filter	How do you use the filter?
Possible potential	The realization of the potential
Exists, but is undeveloped	Intentionally developed

---

[6]   Rath, T. (2007). StrengthsFinder 2.0. New York: Gallup Press.
[7]   Rath, T. (2007). StrengthsFinder 2.0. New York: Gallup Press.

- The goal is to turn each talent into an intentional strength by consciously applying it in your life. In order to do this, you first have to know what your talents are. When you discover and apply them repeatedly, they become tools like knives and forks, and eventually strengths. People have talents naturally—strengths must be developed. Talents are just the foundation for the stress prevention. If you neglect to develop them into strengths, they can cause stress and burnout as well!

- A simple and easy way to develop a talent into a strength is by investing time, knowledge and skills! Compare it with a relationship with a new partner. How will this relationship become solid enough for bigger steps and challenges? You need to get to know the other person—the good and demanding facts; what pleases and displeases them, what are their triggers?

  If you are focused on growing a solid and sustainable relationship, you will need to know more than the superficial facts. This won't be done in a second, you'll need to have persistence, appreciation and faith! Some of the new challenges will need patience and love to work with—others will just be acceptable—and that is just fine. The goal of all of this is to develop the relationship with your new partner into something much bigger—it's worth it. As it is to develop a talent into a strength! Your life will be grounded on a much more solid foundation, and you will reach levels and achieve goals you never thought were possible!

- Clifton Strengths® opens up a new way to understanding your weaknesses and, more importantly, dealing with them. With the awareness of the difference between talent and strengths you have a wonderful tool to manage weaknesses, and the sources of stress and burnout. No one is perfect. This is not what you are here for. With Clifton Strengths® you can start to learn to be perfectly who you are.

- **Here is a list of the 34 Clifton Strengths Talent Themes:**

Achiever®	Deliberative®	Learner®
Activator®	Developer®	Maximizer®
Adaptability®	Discipline®	Positivity®
Analytical®	Empathy®	Relator®
Arranger®	Focus®	Responsibility®
Belief®	Futuristic®	Restorative™
Command®	Harmony®	Self-Assurance®
Communication®	Ideation®	Significance®
Competition®	Includer®	Strategic®
Connectedness®	Individualization®	Woo®
Consistency®	Input®	
Context®	Intellection®	

Clifton Strengths® assessment and the report you'll get after you complete the assessment is the beginning of your journey and the starting point for the ENJOY process!

Again—Clifton Strengths® is the language, while ENJOY is the process to create a plan for a healthier life with the celebration of your own self to prevent unnecessary stress. Are you ready?

CHAPTER 3

The ENJOY Process

Effective stress and burnout prevention is like a mosaic made from many small pieces. It is mainly based on being aware of, and accepting your special and incomparable uniqueness. The first part of the ENJOY process is covered by Clifton Strengths®. Your top 5 talents of Clifton Strengths® are the basis of the ENJOY process and help you find and explain your own personal uniqueness.

What makes you unique? How are you different from the person sitting across from you? Who are you? What do you need to function at your best?

If you don't understand your needs, how are others supposed to understand them? Talents are the filters through which you view the world. They illustrate how you think, communicate, deal with other people, and manage everything in your life. Clifton Strengths® does not tell you what you do, but HOW you do it.

But the ENJOY process is so much more. After you become aware of your own beauty you will explore how you can use "being different" to prevent stress and burnout. Intentionally, you will create a solid comfort zone. Stress and burnout prevention only makes sense when you act from a stable and solid comfort zone. This foundation will be the groundwork of your personal development plan. The ENJOY process is your solid instruction to make sense of all the parts of the mosaic of your life. Let's glue the parts together!

Complete one level of ENJOY after the other to best overcome life's challenges and to take advantage of the opportunities in your life.

E - Embrace Who You Are!

The E in ENJOY stands for "Embrace." Find out who you are and accept your uniqueness. Discover and embrace your comfort zone, and how best to use it.

In this first step of ENJOY, you will learn what is unique about you and why you should be extremely proud of yourself. At the same time, the E in ENJOY is the most important step. It is the foundation of all work that will come after this point. A house cannot exist for long without a solid base.

You are born with a different combination of talents. Nobody sees the world exactly the way you do. If you don't know your talents or how to use them, they become weaknesses or stressors. They can become a problem for you, as well as others.

If you try to suppress one of your talents or if you don't like it, it is like a cast on your arm or leg—you cannot use the affected limb. In this situation, you would not use these body parts intentionally. You can best acknowledge your talents when you understand how much they have helped you realize your goals and dreams in the past. Learn to understand how each individual strength influences your thoughts, feelings, and behaviors.

Everyone has an exclusive combination of talents. This unique combination of talents is what gives you the potential to be world class in one area. But you need talent as a main prerequisite to be able to develop a true strength and become world class. By investing time and by deepening your knowledge of a talent, you can gradually develop a true strength. This strength becomes the solid foundation for your comfort zone. Therefore, it is the basis for lasting stress and burnout prevention. Only when you embrace your talents, can you become a world class champion!

Maybe this image will help you: think about 5 acquaintances. These are people you know but are not terribly close to. They are existent—and that's it. Can you trust them? Would you welcome them with open arms and hugs and kisses? Not really, right? In order to do so you want to know more about them, know what you can expect from them, understand when they can be there for you. Step by step, a relationship will be developed.

This is exactly the kind of relationship you want to have with your talents. You want to get to know them; no restrictions, no distance, no rejection. Instead you should feel adoration, joy, and love for them. The E of the ENJOY process will help you transform acquaintances into soulmates. Understand and embrace your talents and who you are.

N - Nurture: Stress Prevention

In the first step of ENJOY, you have gained insight into what exactly your talents are, the importance these talents have had in your life, and why it only makes sense to love them.

Now, learn to use this insight and nurture your talents for stress prevention here, in the second step, **N**. Yes, it really is as simple as that. You have everything in you to prevent stress taking over your life. Not all at once, because it will take you some time to nurture your talents into real strengths.

And, even after you are aware of them and can use them to your advantage on a daily basis, you are still a human being with good and bad days. Some days it will be easier to nurture and use your talents. But, if you had a long day or if you didn't get enough sleep, you'll face moments where it is going to be more difficult to embrace and nurture the awareness of your talents into your thought process.

Sometimes, it's all we can do to get through the day in one piece, and that's okay. Start fresh the next day and remember to embrace and nurture you, because you are what matters most.

The aspect of nurturing is crucial. How can you feed and develop your talents? It's kind of like having a baby bird in your nest—until the baby bird is ready to survive on its own, you have to feed it with the right amount of food it needs to grow. The nutrition for growing and nurturing your talents is something that depends on each one of your talent themes.

Once you understand what exactly is unique about you, you will soon also know what you need in order to work effectively. Conversely, if you have not met these prerequisites, you will develop stress factors.

With **N**, you can learn how to curb or prevent these stress factors. Use your uniqueness and nurture your talents into strengths to protect yourself against stress.

J - Jump into YOUR System

In the first 2 steps of ENJOY, **E** and **N**, you've learned to embrace and nurture your natural talents. You've built the most important foundations for stress prevention. Now, in **J**, we move on to design your unique plan for stress and burnout prevention. It's time to jump into a new routine and system that is designed just for you. Get ready, get set, now JUMP!

You cannot expect a change unless you facilitate one. This is why I call it "Jump". It's like standing at the edge of the swimming pool, taking a deep breath, and jumping in! We're not talking about wading in from the steps here. Jump and create a plan that will help you to carry out your personalized ENJOY process.

This plan has to be based on your own needs and talents. Review old patterns, move your body and brain and start over! I know it's hard, I'll give you a push if you need it! To help you replace old entrenched patterns with new promising patterns, you need YOUR PLAN (my push, if you will). This plan includes routines and habits you first must establish—so that they work for you—and you then have to incorporate them deliberately into your everyday life.

By this, I mean routines and habits related to your body as well as your thought process; move your brain and your body. The old system was not effective. Jump into YOUR new system, with your talents in mind.

O - Optimize

Successful stress prevention becomes effective when you align and optimize yourself in relation to your talents. Based on your talent themes, a new routine, fixed and designed in the plan we started in **J**, will help you pave the way for effective stress prevention.

It is essential to incorporate sleep and nutrition into your routine. And, an approach on how to manage your time and yourself in ways that work for you. Awareness must take place on all levels. You jumped into your new life in **J—O** will now help you to optimize your system as you need it. You develop this system—your plan, step by step—starting with Clifton Strengths®. Continue to create habits and routines to have a long-term success.

Y - YOU

The cherry on the I of ENJOY is the conscious and loving examination of the self—You. With **Y**, you'll add mindfulness and breathing techniques to your plan—and you'll use your new self-awareness to wrap up your ENJOY process. Sharpen the saw, round the edges. Get your plan as effective as possible and start to aim your new skills and awareness towards the outside. It's time to take it from ME to WE.

After all, you are the most important part of your ENJOY process—**Y** within ENJOY is synonymous with a "period" at the end of a sentence. You are responsible for your actions, behaviors and your life. No one else.

As I mentioned earlier, it's best to complete the ENJOY process in the order listed above. Each step of the process—**E, N, J, O,** and **Y**—builds on the one before it. You can't nurture your talents before you learn to embrace them.

ENJOY—for whom?

For Each and Every One of You

Clifton Strengths® will change the world. The thought of what will happen once everyone knows his/her own strengths fascinates and enthralls me. It is so optimistic. People around the globe finally have the chance to understand themselves and others.

It is as if the world suddenly had a new language that can be understood by EVERYONE. You will be able to communicate on a whole new level. Stress will occur on a new level and mental health will be redefined.

Regardless of race, origin, sexual orientation, male or female ... everything can be redefined. The purpose of my approach is to give courage. To give hope. To motivate and inspire the development of different ideas.

The ENJOY process is your plan to lean on and translate the new knowledge you gained with Clifton Strengths® in every area of your life. A plan with routines tailored to make you the most successful and healthiest person you can be. ENJOY contributes to how you interact with others, now and in the future, how and who you are.

For Companies and Organizations.

The reason I became a coach is that I could not bear to see how some people treat each other in their professional, as well as in their private lives. There is often not a lot of appreciation for others. Instead, everybody only tries to get ahead—in most cases, regardless of the consequences, intentionally or unintentionally.

Often, lack of self-esteem or self-appreciation is the root cause. Many people have never learned or seen anything different. I wanted to change this, I wanted my work to impact how people interact with each other in their professional lives.

The ENJOY process will support the challenges senior management is currently facing. The expectations placed on senior management and managers are changing rapidly. It is no longer enough to merely be the boss. A manager or team leader must also have the right tools to be credible and accepted, to be authentic, and to be a role model. It is not only about the hierarchy within the company that defines the roles and the knowledge of a manager, there is more cooperation.

This in turn, requires senior managers to develop true management skills. These not only include leadership knowledge and skills, but above all the ability to be human. How can somebody be a leader and at the same time be human? With ENJOY, we begin to introduce a new management culture in companies and organizations. A management culture based on human uniqueness.

Employees who feel understood and appreciated are healthier, do not want to leave the company, support the boss with all they can do, and are less stressed. It is reflected in the fact that you see the beaming faces of your employees, hear the laughter in the halls of your offices, and that your employees truly trust you. The statistics of customer satisfaction, revenues, and the decreasing costs for hiring new employees will speak for themselves.

ENJOY is the most effective and healthy foundation for every company, but above all, it is the perfect process for long-lasting stress and burnout prevention.

ENJOY will allow any organization and team to embrace human uniqueness, become a strengths-based organization AND accept wholeheartedly the responsibility that comes with the position of its leaders and managers.

Leadership will be elevated to a new level. Management can concentrate on their actual role: planning the company's future and the strategic direction in order to face challenges. This saves time and energy that was constantly needed for crisis management and personnel problems before.

A new corporate culture with ENJOY will redefine the entire image of the company.

CHAPTER 4

What We Know So Far

Known Facts ...

Stress

The word "stress" alone, causes stress in a lot of people because it plays a large role in their lives. Because they know what stress feels like. And above all, because they know what affect stress has in their lives. Stress alone is not a bad thing of course—there is positive stress. Since you have no idea how you are supposed to deal with it, the word has a largely negative connotation.

The other reason is that many people know that stress is present in the unconscious way before it is noticed. Some people may know how to deal with stress, have read books, or taken classes. Nothing has really helped—which causes even more stress—because this makes you feel vulnerable and powerless.

You experience stress when basic needs or different key factors are not met. These are some of the key factors and basic needs that may influence people's wellbeing and their stress level:

- Income and social status
- Social support
- Education and literacy
- Employment/working conditions
- Social environment
- Physical conditions
- Individual ways to stay healthy
- Good preconditions for kids to grow up healthy
- Biological and genetic preconditions
- Hygiene
- Gender
- Culture

It doesn't matter if you live in South Africa or Germany, depending on what your brain has stored as "normal" you experience danger and stress on different levels. If your basic needs are not met, the fight or flight response kicks in—and the body has no choice but to react and help you to survive.

Originally, stress was designed to help people survive; nothing more and nothing less. Its origin therefore dates back over 2,000 years. Back then, it was a mere matter of survival. The world has evolved—but not the foundation of your brain. Your brain works exactly as it did 2,000 years ago! Stress helped you to escape and save your life. You may not still be running from predators but, you are still running!

Therefore, stress is completely normal, it continues to save your life. It enables you to accomplish things you never thought possible. You react faster, run faster, breathe faster, and are much more alert.

Here is a list of indications your body gives you when it experiences stress. You may not even attribute some of them to stress—but they have the same effect on your body. Are you familiar with these indicators?

- Recurring headaches/teeth grinding
- Cold and clammy hands and feet
- Trouble breathing
- Sighing frequently and dry mouth
- Problems swallowing
- Stuttering or stammering
- Shaking, wobbly knees
- Neck pain, "back", muscle tensions
- Dizziness, unease, sweating
- Ringing in the ears, "popping" in the ears
- Susceptible to common colds, infections, frequent herpes
- Skin rash and itching / unexplained allergies
- Stomach aches, unease
- Extreme bloating and diarrhea
- Panic attacks, increased heart rate, chest pain
- Excessive suspiciousness
- Social withdrawal and isolation
- Constantly tired, worn-out, and burned out
- Increased consumption of light "drugs"
- Unusually high addiction to gambling
- Shopaholic
- Frequent urination
- Low sex drive
- Nervousness, anxieties, feelings of guilt
- More annoyed, frustrated, bad mood
- Depression, constant mood changes
- Increased or decreased appetite

- Trouble sleeping, nightmares
- Trouble and difficulties – concentrating
- Chaotic thoughts and learning difficulties, forgetfulness, confusion
- No or reduced decision-making capability
- Overwhelmed by feelings, crying fits
- Feeling of loneliness and without self-worth
- Not attaching any importance on appearance and punctuality
- Increased frustration, irritability, overreaction to small details
- Minor accidents, reduced work productivity
- Lying and making excuses to cover up poor work
- Mumbling

The human body is a miracle—and it works wonders. If you experience stress, there is the Autonomous Nervous System (ATS) to protect you—and your body reacts.

I don't want to annoy you with facts about the exact reactions, there are enough books and information out there to study this if you'd like more detail.

Just let me tell you, that our wonderful ATS, divided into the Sympathetic Nervous system (SNS) and Parasympathetic Nervous System (PNS), will decide—depending on the signals and signs from your body (danger or peace) how to react. Whether you want it to or not, this is out of your control. Before you even realize it, the autopilot ATS guides you and your reactions. You feel stressed—maybe super stressed!

That means, you must take control and react before this happens. But how?

Permanent Stress

Being permanently in the fight and flight mode will guide you into permanent stress mode—the perfect launching point for burnout. Permanent stress means your body has no downtime to relax and recharge its batteries for the next challenge. And there will be a next challenge! Life is all about the challenges, and they will keep coming as long as you are alive! You are born to face them!

Burnout

But here is the point! Usually you are not aware when you are in permanent stress, because this won't happen from one second to the next. Everything is connected! It starts slowly as stress and becomes more and more ... and at some point, you may be hit by a burnout. Burnout is a message from your body, telling you that you ran several red lights where it tried to explain to you to change something. But these red lights have been ignored.

This is how your system actually works. Continue your life, continue ignoring your uniqueness and do what others tell you —add a few prevention techniques—and you'll be fine! You have to be. If not, there is someone else waiting for your job.

The experience I've gained from working with clients is that the body has indeed sent various warning signals. However, they were not recognized or they were ignored in fear of having to make changes. A complete breakdown finally ensures that you must think about what is actually going on. As crazy as it sounds, it is a protection mechanism of the body that is designed to ensure that you get well again.

Permanent stress and burnout are not under your control anymore! You have to understand this! It's way too late to use stress and burnout prevention techniques once you are in a stressful situation or maybe even experiencing permanent stress. And way too late if you have been hit by a burnout. Prevention will not help at this point.

Now, reflect for a second. Are you on the path to experience the joy of a burnout?

12 Phases According to Freudenberger

Herbert Freudenberger[8] and his colleague Gail North, identified twelve phases you go through in the course of burnout syndrome. They outlined them as (order does not matter):

1. The urge to prove something to ourselves and others.

2. Need for achievement and the necessity to meet especially high expectations.

3. Working too much while neglecting personal needs and social contacts.

4. Covering up or ignoring personal problems and conflicts.

5. Doubting our own system of values as well as neglecting things that used to be important to us such as hobbies and friends.

6. Denial of emerging problems, lowering of the tolerance limit.

7. Withdrawing and avoiding social contacts.

8. Obvious behavior changes, increasing feeling of worthlessness, growing anxiety.

---

[8] Freudenberger,H. & North,G. (Freiburg, 1992)

9. Depersonalization due to loss of contact with ourselves and other people; life becomes increasingly automated and mechanical.

10. Feeling of emptiness and desperate attempts to cover up these feelings through things like sex, eating, alcohol, or drugs.

11. Depression with symptoms such as indifference, hopelessness, fatigue, and lack of perspective.

12. Thoughts of suicide as a way to escape the situation; acute risk of a mental and/or physical breakdown.

How we used to approach stress is not working, we need a new approach; way before permanent stress becomes our best partner and friend. Before stress and burnout prevention techniques become just another way for some coaches to earn money or a way managers can spend part of their health budgets and feel good about themselves.

The way the system continues down the old paths leaves me speechless. **Because this is intentional gross bodily injury.** Stress is a life saver, and continues to be abused again and again by wrong behavior. And most people are not even aware of it, because, otherwise, would they not treat their body differently, right?

Or in the words of Martha Graham, in her book, *Blood Memory*[9], "The body is a sacred garment. It's your first and your last garment; it's what you enter life in and what you depart life with, and it should be treated with honor, and with joy and with fear as well. But always, though, with blessing."

If you constantly disregard and misuse your body, you shouldn't be surprised when there are consequences—burnout!

---

[9] Graham, M. (1991). Blood memory. New York: Doubleday.

CHAPTER 5

Reality Check #1

Stress, Anxiety and Depression are caused
when we are living to please others.

(Paul Coelho)

Paula, James, Isabelle, and Adam—four wonderful people, all of them well-educated, who virtually have all the information available to prevent them from falling into the burnout trap. All of them asked themselves "HOW?" They apparently did not see, or did not want to accept the facts. Or could they not see it because the perception of society does not allow it?

You are not allowed to appear weak. The basic principle still applies that, regardless of how many positive talents you have, the main thing is to recognize your weaknesses and to work on them so they can be eliminated. But this is the main reason for stress. If you do not live and embrace your talents ... you get stressed.

I want to use these wonderful people to show you the correlations. They are not based on scientific findings. Any university professor who feels inspired by my ideas may want to research all of this scientifically.

The personal history of people, their behavior, and the reactions people get, as a result of their behavior, are all interrelated. You can see this if you take a step back. However, in most cases you do not have or take the time to recognize these correlations. Sometimes, this is because you are in pain, tired, or sad, or sometimes it is simply to protect yourself. The fact is that you could learn a lot from real life experiences. What stops you?

Four wonderful human beings who ignored their red lights! These individuals explained their situation in their own words, and gave me the chance to better illustrate my theory based on their experiences, feelings, and observations. Read their stories:

Paula

Paula was a very successful project manager at a large German company. Through adult education, she finished high school at the top of her class, studied economics at the University of Cologne, where she also finished at the top of her class. She started a promising career and had a lot of fun and success at first.

Her supervisor was a good manager, saw her potential, and gave her the freedom she needed to be successful. He therefore created the basis for ensuring that Paula went home happy at the end of the day, because she felt that she was at the right place with her skills. She was recognized for her commitment and was well respected for her good performance, but also for her personality.

However, she then got a new supervisor. Not everything changed—but a number of things did. The most important thing was that her freedom was taken away from her (at least this is how she felt) and she was no longer allowed to be directly responsible for the work she did. Being controlled left her no room to breathe. Every day, she felt like she was climbing into a cage where all happiness, light, and sun was taken away from her. She began having physical problems, which were minor at first, but then become increasingly severe.

The end of this apparent success story is that Paula went to the Human Resources Manager and explained the situation. In the meantime, she had been to the emergency room two times and was barely able to stand up straight because of cramps. Her gastrointestinal tract and other organs quit working properly. Not even 40 years old, her body pulled the emergency brake as well. Nothing was working properly anymore.

The Human Resources Manager did not have the language to understand Paula's needs. And Paula could not explain what she needed in order to do her best every day. Paula was lucky that the company wanted to restructure anyway and let her go with a compensation.

She left the company with the stale feeling of having failed. She only saw what she did not accomplish, what did not work. There were plenty of young managers eager for a career standing by to take over her job.

Paula had what it takes for this job but, it still was not enough. Her body told her where her limit was. What happened?

Adam

Adam was a successful engineer... but ... not happy and he was stressed. He was a cheerful boy when he left school at the age of 15 to start an apprenticeship as a skilled electrician. But he sensed early on during his apprenticeship, that this was not the career path he wanted to pursue until his retirement, he wanted more.

So, he decided to continue his education and study electrical engineering. Over the years, he became increasingly fascinated with cars. It was only natural for him to apply to a large automotive manufacturer after getting his engineering degree, where he started his career with a lot of enthusiasm.

Adam was able to make his dreams a reality and was hired because of his education, experience, and motivation. And the first years went well, very well in fact. The reputation of his employer was dazzling, the products he supported were awesome, and the prestige of his work among his friends let Adam float on clouds. He had in fact achieved a lot.

However, he noticed as time went by that something was not right, both in his private life as well as in his job. Was this really the life he had dreamed about?

At work, he realized that the daily waste of material of the automotive industry, and the way of working together no longer matched his ideals. In the meantime, Adam worked in Quality Assurance. Day in and day out, he was busy keeping the quality of his employer's products at the highest level possible, or finding solutions for suddenly emerging problems.

His zest for life disappeared. Everyday life was mainly centered around problems and complaints. The splendor and the emotion for vehicles and the fascination for the technology faded away from year to year. He was barely able to use his own strengths. The spiral of frustration had started to turn, even before he realized it and now started to turn faster and faster.

Adam was still able to push reality from his mind. The head-in-the-sand tactics carried him through the days and weeks. He simply did not want to accept what was already clearly visible from the outside. There were a lot of good friends as well as family members who kept telling him that he could not continue at this level of pressure. Others realized what he could not.

Unfortunately, he ignored them all. He noticed that he could no longer pursue his passion for cooking and had no more free time. But ambition carried him along for some time—until he could no longer continue.

On a weekend shortly before Easter, he fell into a bottomless void. Almost 72 hours without sleep; thousands of random pictures that appeared before his eyes every second. No distraction was able to stop this jumble of pictures.

That was it—he had reached his limit, his body sent clear signals. He was burnt out. Now he could no longer continue. Friends and family urged Adam to see a doctor for help. The doctor threw his hands up in exasperation and sent him on sick leave. What happened?

Isabelle

Isabelle's story is completely different. As a child, she grew up in the countryside and spent a lot of time in nature. Her parents supported her, but at the same time taught her that we are only valuable if we achieve something. This is why after high school and a dual major, she quickly climbed the corporate ladder.

In her mid-twenties, she was already working 50 to 60-hour weeks. Isabelle did not even intend to advance as quickly as she did. The truth was that she was not able to see her own limits—she had forgotten to pay attention to herself and her needs.

Her neglect for herself and her own personal needs, resulted in a severe illness a few years later, which forced her to change her thinking. After spending four weeks in a hospital and the same amount of time in rehab, she quit her job and took some time off. Her loving partner, who had been by her side for a number of years already, made this possible.

The years passed, Isabelle now had three kids and was in her mid-thirties. She started to feel that there was more to life and started a career in healthcare. She became successful there as well. So much so that her body went on strike after eight years.

The double pressure: juggling a family, household, and job were more than she could handle. She felt drained, empty, and was not able to think clearly. Her zest for life was gone. She slept in on weekends but still felt tired and broken afterwards. Everything hurt—she was burnt out as well. And this despite the fact, or maybe precisely because, she worked in healthcare? What happened?

James

James was a successful bank production manager in Frankfurt. Happily married, with one child, very well integrated socially in a small Hessian town. Like many employees in the Rhine-Main region, he made the 2-hour train ride to Frankfurt every day to be able to get to his workplace in the banking hub. He was sharp, intelligent, and very dedicated. He was a group manager and his supervisors were very happy with him.

Due to his skills, he quickly rose up in the ranks, had a large number of projects simultaneously or one after the other. James was a workaholic who was always assigned with yet another project because he was so reliable. It became increasingly difficult to balance day-to-day operations, as well as project and personnel management.

It was in his nature to complete a task very conscientiously. This was not only the case at work—but also at home. He was very active in various clubs in his hometown because of his parents' commitment. He was reliable: When James had a job, when friends asked him for help, he was there and, he didn't quit until the work was done. Barely back home from work, he continued right away. And he had always done it that way; it became his routine.

He started getting viral infections regularly, developed high blood pressure, and was often irritable and tired. Then he started to lose his appetite. He developed insomnia. His heart was racing and did not let him settle down. At some point, he went to the doctor. An ECG and other tests did not reveal anything—the doctor advised him to eat healthy, lose weight, and slow down a little. He also motivated him to exercise more.

But all in all, everything continued as before. He continued to feel like a hamster in a wheel. Adding exercise into his daily schedule only added more stress.

Then, one day, he could not do it anymore. On a Saturday, James had only wanted to visit his wife at a trade fair, nothing worked any more. After he arrived at the parking lot, he could not get out of the car. He had a complete shutdown. His body drew a line—pulled the emergency brake—that James had not wanted to pull himself. BURNOUT. What happened?

CHAPTER 6

Cause & Effect

Root Cause Analysis

● We are Not Aware of Our Uniqueness

You are born a small miracle. A miracle because it is still incomprehensible how the first two cells eventually developed into something as perfect as a little baby. Children have been born for thousands of years. Whether they are loved or not loved, planned or not planned, protected or not protected. They are born—and from the beginning, it is about survival.

What does a person need to become **somebody**? For what purpose was this person born? How many parents know that these little creatures should not be confronted immediately with what is expected of them? How many children are given the chance to fulfill their purpose in life? Each individual born on this earth has his/her own way of communicating, approaching challenges, selecting projects, and figuring out their own likes and dislikes. You are exclusive. Ignoring this leads to stress.

• Comparisons

One of the root causes of stress is comparisons. You compare large and small apples, apples and oranges, peppers and pineapple, it never ends. After a child is born, you first compare which one is larger or stronger. Sometimes, it makes sense to compare. However, the result of comparisons can leave others disillusioned.

In business, a comparison might result in further development; which is definitely a positive thing.

Some people also need this; they constantly need to have the opportunity to compare themselves to others. The Competition® talent theme of Clifton Strengths® describes this very idea. These people measure their own progress on the achievements of others. They are inspired by comparison. But, we are not all the same.

Comparisons have a negative effect on performance level and achievement potential, they crush and demotivate—and therefore cause stress—factors which lead to burnout.

• Incorrect Priorities

People have basic needs. Abraham Maslow[10] (1908-1970) illustrated them in his hierarchy of needs. Stress develops if these basic needs are not met. However, some of the most basic needs can be neglected when you forget the self—the things that make you unique. In Maslow's theory, self-actualization is at the top of the pyramid. Instead, satisfying your own needs and developing your talents should be at the foundation of the hierarchy. If you do not satisfy this need, you feel stressed.

---

[10]   Maslow, A.H. (1943). "A Theory of Human Motivation". In *Psychological Review*, 50 (4), 430-437. Washington, DC: American Psychological Association. 013

● Fight for the Ideal Job

Another reason why you experience stress is your desire to have the best job in the world. From an early age, you are taught that the only thing that is important in life is the highest paying job you can get. Regardless of your own unique talents and skills, our society encourages you to sacrifice everything, in order to get a job with the highest salary or the loftiest reputation.

If this means that you have to move or travel—it does not matter. All that matters is that you get the job. For many people, a job is the key to happiness; money, wealth, prestige. Even if you cannot realize your own potential—the only thing that matters is the ideal job. You tend to compete for the ideal job—but not for your job! This is a huge trigger for stress.

● Improper Distribution of Tasks

If you don't know what makes you unique and what your special talents and strengths are, you do not have the self-assurance to demand what you need to thrive. This causes a lack of communication which, in turn makes it impossible to properly distribute tasks within a group of people.

The people who dare to speak up are once again the winners. The ones s who have difficulties stepping into the light are the losers here—even though they often would be better suited to complete these tasks. This starts a cycle—improper task distribution creates an imbalance and causes stress among everyone involved.

● Lack of Management Skills

Your company culture lacks leaders and coaches. Employees are told what they are supposed to do. Often, they don't know the why and they are missing the support and knowledge that they are contributors to the success of the organization.

Employees often can only accept the situation and try not to fall from grace. Quitting their job is the only way out. If employees don't have great managers…. then the longest list of perks is not going to be a cure-all.[11] According to polls from Gallup, more than 50% of all employees leave their company because of their manager. The lack of management skills first leads to stress—and maybe to more stress to find new employees.

I'm sure there are a lot more possible reasons to create stress. But, what they all have in common is that embracing the human uniqueness would eliminate almost, if not all of these causes for stress.

Effects of Stress and Burnout

Stress and Burnout effect each one of you on so many levels.

• Individual

Life is going to be very different after a burnout. It's huge—the message burnout gives us is—change something, change the way you approached life, organized your comfort zone. Change yourself! Loud and clear— this is the message!

• Professional

Even on the professional level, stress and burnout will have a huge impact. It will take a while after a burnout to come back. With the wrong

---

[11] GALLUP, State of the American Workplace, (2017)

perception that often comes with a burnout, you would lose trust in yourself and your capabilities.

With a powerful new approach and an understanding why the burnout happened, you could start over. You often do not have the opportunity to resume at the point in your career where you left off before the breakdown. But, this may be just right!

• Financial

This point may have been the main reason for you to push through the permanent stress before the burnout—financial insecurity. This effect may be the factor scaring you the most. You need money to live. After the breakdown, everything may be different. You have to readjust and rearrange your life. Usually you tend to avoid big changes but, this change has to be accepted.

• Society

According to worldwide health report[12], illnesses that are caused by psychological problems are increasing significantly. Therefore, the costs for these types of illnesses are increasing, as well.

And it is an illusion if you think that the costs for missing work after a burnout are not incurred until after the day the employee is no longer coming to work. In one of my clients, clear signs of severe depression were already recognizable 2 years in advance. This means that employees are only working at perhaps 70% of their potential, probably even a lot less, before their actual absence. They are a lot more susceptible to colds and back problems than "healthy" individuals.

---

[12]   BKK Gesundheitsreport (2015), TK Gesundheitsreport (2011), World Health Organisation

And with the shadow, stress and burnout spread all over the world, the fear of failure and health issues gets bigger and bigger. People are not capable of being effective and successful unless they are confident and strong in what they do—and who they are. The effects of stress and burnout will become unmanageable. As I said earlier—we need a change!

CHAPTER 7

Reality Check #2

Paula

For Paula, this was not the end of the world. Like I said, Paula had received a compensation that made it possible for her to maintain financial stability. She became self-employed, started an agency, and developed web pages for clients. Not too bad—but she was left with the feeling of having failed. She had worked at one of the leading companies in Germany and was not able to cope with the pressure.

She often doubted herself, she was frustrated, and sad. Should it not have been possible to go on longer, was she a coward? It should have been possible somehow. This way of thinking did not help nor promote her sense of self-worth. The gastrointestinal problems slowly disappeared, but what remained was the deep mental wound.

Paula is still suffering from the after-effects to this day. And they will probably continue for quite a while, if they ever disappear altogether.

Adam

Confronted with the reality that he had been running away from for much too long, Adam only wanted to get away, simply get away. He needed time and space to be able to get lost in his thoughts in a relaxed atmosphere to understand what had happened. Why and when did he stop taking himself seriously enough to give everything else a higher priority?

After 8 weeks, he returned to his old company with the clear intention of not slipping back into old habits. Before his time off, he had talked to his supervisor. He told him very clearly that he would not continue as before. His supervisor had promised him to change these conditions by restructuring the department. But the system in the organization was not flexible enough. Then Adam made his decision.

He went to Human Resources and reduced his work week to 30 hours; he cut back to working only 4 days a week. He wanted to use his day off to build on and apply his talents, something that was not promoted or valued in his job. Talents he could only apply to a very limited extent at work.

What he had realized was that he was increasingly confronted with being told what to do. His own natural talents were not taken account nor recognized at all. Adam is a person who has a lot of ideas and thinks outside the box. This could not be used in his daily work.

He started to use his creativity to create something new—something beautiful. He founded a start-up company. The first project of this company was supposed to be a bathroom series made from concrete.

From the design on the desk to the finished end product, he made everything himself on his "day off." He created his own logo and web page. He also started going to trade fairs to talk about his creations and publicize them.

He was finally able to be himself. His life finally started to have meaning in a way he was not able to grasp before. It felt absolutely amazing to experience how the various strengths all of a sudden helped in a fun way to put such a project on a sound foundation.

Adam recognized that burnout was the result of driving past too many red lights. The body did not know any other way to help itself. Burnout was the end of a dead-end street. What could have been different?

Isabelle

Once again, she was forced to change something in her life. She realized that family is one of her most important values that had to be preserved. Isabelle used her strengths yet again to come out of this low point. She gathered information, learned everything about burnout, and even trained to become a burnout coach.

Life sometimes takes strange turns ... a new illness let Isabelle recognize that she is only at her best when she integrates and uses all of her strengths.

James

Life led James directly to the clinic. He was admitted to a hospital, initially stabilized with psychiatric drugs, but then sent home because there was no space available. With a bit of luck, he got a bed in a clinic after 6 weeks to slowly get him back on track.

He was released after 8 weeks of treatment but, was far from being ready to return to work. Weeks, months after his breakdown, he started returning to his old job again slowly, but under different conditions—very slowly.

Today, James works a full 40 hours a week again. His managers were very understanding of his situation. One of the reasons being that the department had already lost 3 employees due to psychosomatic illness before James. In some cases, the consequences were much more severe than they were for James.

James learned to emphasize his talents and prioritize activities correspondingly. He understood himself better, was better able to articulate his needs to other people, especially to his supervisors, which made it easier for him to say NO if necessary.

CHAPTER 8

ENJOY in Your Life - The Process

E -Embrace

Get yourself ready for a journey through the ENJOY process. You are about to learn to recognize and embrace the traits that make you perfect and how best to use them to protect yourself from feeling stressed, frustrated and unhappy. Ready? Here we go:

Embrace Who You Are!

Your natural talents are the basis for being truly successful. They are your comfort zone! They ensure that you feel self-confident and secure. If you are in your comfort zone, you are courageous and creative; it is easy for you to excel here. This reassurance is a relief. The parasympathetic nervous system helps you relax so that you have access to all the information in your brain. You are calm and composed, you radiate authenticity, and attract people who want to support you in what you want to achieve. This is the best possible starting point in all respects.

Stress occurs when you want to achieve the impossible by any means necessary. It is easiest to achieve excellence in the areas where you inherent, natural talent. But how do you recognize these areas?

This is why the first and most important step is to be able to name and explain YOUR talents. **Embrace who you are** with **E.**

I will use this chapter to help you understand how you can start this ENJOY process for yourself. I will use one of my clients as an example and explain how my ENJOY process supported her very effectively in her daily life.

A successful collaboration between a client and myself or between you and ENJOY starts with Clifton Strengths®. The online assessment is the prerequisite before we even start with the ENJOY process. You can find the online Clifton Strengths® assessment at www.gallupstrengthscenter.com. You can also find the link on my homepage at www.strengths4you.com.

After you have taken your test, thoroughly read the definitions of the talent themes provided by Gallup in your reports. The general definition of your top 5 talents as you can find it in the Signature Themes Report. Take a marker and highlight the words and sentences with which you identify—this applies to me, this is who I am. Explore yourself openly and honestly.

When are you most successful, what are you doing? What are you doing in these types of instances? Which actions empower you? When can you say, "Yes, this is who I am. Yes, this is how I can see myself."? Get to know your strengths and become aware of how you can help yourself and others when you use these talents.

Or, you may decide to give the report to someone who knows you; someone you are close to. Ask this person to use a different color to mark how they see you. This provides some very interesting feedback as well.

The more you know what YOUR talents are and how these talents can help you and others be more successful, the easier it will be for you to acknowledge them and stop admiring the talents of others. You direct the focus inwards! This is the beginning of true growth. Every breath you take and every move you make, everything is controlled by your talents.

Clifton Strengths® provides us with the areas where we have the greatest potential. Even though it is very important to know this—it will only help you to a limited extent to get ahead and become truly successful. The goal is to turn our talents into real strengths and to then use them to prevent stress and burnout. This takes time, knowledge, and patience.

The result of Clifton Strengths® is a powerful list of your natural talents. But with no action your report remains just that—simply a list! It is only a start. As described earlier, it is your responsibility to transform your talents into strengths. **E – Embrace your talents.** The more you incorporate these talents into your everyday life and use them deliberatively, the faster you will develop these talents into strengths.

These strengths will help you grow as a person and to increase your personal performance tremendously. This individual growth creates your comfort zone. Each of your dominant talents is a key to a life of self-assurance, well-being, uniqueness, and pride.

At the same time, knowing and being aware of your talents will help you manage your weaknesses. A weakness is simply a misapplication of talent, skill or knowledge and could cause problems for you or for others. Your ability to deliberately deal with your talents will help you manage these weaknesses. You are human. You will never be perfect. But developing your talents will help you become the absolute best you can be!

You have your combination of talents; they are unique and precious. Others have their wonderful combination of talents as well. They are very valuable for the world as well. No single talent is more precious or more important than any of the others.

Yes, we have a framework: Clifton Strengths® and all 34 talent themes are included. You need all talent themes to get a homogeneous structure. It makes absolutely no sense to rate the individual categories or talent themes and say "this one is more important than the other." It would create limits that prevent us from being able to tap the full potential of the talent themes. Alone nothing is possible, together everything is possible.

You were created to overcome challenges together. When you give a rating, you once again come to the conclusion that some people are more important than others. This is nonsense because you need different talents on different occasions. Nobody is perfect and we need each and every one of us to create a beautiful world and to keep it that way. What a great fact! We need each other.

Simply start to get to know your true self. Expand your comfort zone to create the prerequisite for effective stress prevention.

Be bold and courageous, learn to listen to yourself and not what "others" are saying about you or to you. Why should others' opinions be more valid than what you feel and see for yourself? It is time to put yourself and your own thoughts first because what is the worst thing that can happen? You live, you find out who you are, and finally leave your own footprints on this planet instead of following in the footprints others have left.

Sarah

I want to introduce you to Sarah. She is a successful Michigan business woman who is running her own business and, hired me to help her become more balanced in her life. Her daily routine presented her with challenges—which was ok with her—but she knew she could achieve so much more if she didn't feel constantly stressed throughout her day. Sarah has the following combination of Clifton Strengths® Talent Themes:

TOP 5	TALENT THEME	WHAT IS SPECIAL ABOUT THIS TALENT?
1	Ideation®	People exceptionally talented in the Ideation® theme are fascinated by ideas. They are able to find connection between seemingly disparate phenomena.
2	Adaptability®	People exceptionally talented in the Adaptability® theme prefer to go with the flow. They tend to be "now" people who take things as they come and discover the future one day at a time.
3	Belief®	People exceptionally talented in the Belief® theme have certain core values that are unchanging. Out of these values emerges a defined purpose for their lives.
4	Relator®	People exceptionally talented in the Relator® theme enjoy close relationships with others. They find deep satisfaction in working hard with friends to achieve a goal.

TOP 5	TALENT THEME	WHAT IS SPECIAL ABOUT THIS TALENT?
5	Achiever®	People exceptionally talented in the Achiever® theme work hard and possess a great deal of stamina. They take immense satisfaction in being busy and productive.

The first step for her was to really understand her own personal top 5 talent themes. How are these talent themes explaining her personality?

After completing the online assessment, she started with the first exercise of reading and highlighting her Clifton Strengths® reports. We continued with some general questions about herself. Remember, this stage of the ENJOY process should help her understand her own unique beauty that she has and can share with others. Nothing is just one dimensional. To understand the bigger picture, it is necessary to gather as much information as you can get your hands on. The more curious you become about yourself the better it is! Here are some of the questions we started with:

Ideation®:

- Are you fascinated by ideas and thinking outside the box?
- When are you the most creative and inventive?
- How do you support your need for creativity?
- How do you see this talent theme showing up for you?

Adaptability®:

- When was your greatest moment of change?
- How do you accept challenges and what helps you to live in the here and now?
- What kind of surprises do you embrace and when are you extremely flexible?
- How do you see this talent theme showing up for you?

Belief®:

- How do you create trust with the unchanging presence of your values?
- What are your always present values that serve as your inner compass?
- Do you remember a moment when a decision based on your values helped you to be successful?
- How do you see this talent theme showing up for you?

Relator®:

- What would your best friend say about the kind of friendship you have?
- Are trust and reliability very important values for you?
- What kind of feeling do you have achieving something together with friends?
- How do you see this talent theme showing up for you?

Achiever®:

- What was the biggest project you accomplished because of your tireless and extremely ambitious approach when it comes to work?
- Do you enjoy to get things done and have a work output like a machine?
- Do you need usually any external motivation?
- How do you see this talent theme showing up for you?

In order to help Sarah to see that her talents are her most powerful resources to ENJOY life to the fullest, she needed to see the power behind her talents. *How do Sarah's special combination of talents support her to achieve her goals and successes?*

Her talents are nothing special to her because they are part of who she is. But how can she intentionally use these special gifts in her life, if she is not aware of how special they really are? Walking baby steps, she got more and more inspired by just how much her talents had supported her in her past to achieve excellent successes. And even more impressive for her was the realization that she had lots of fun and felt comfortable while being successful —the opposite of feeling stressed.

This was a huge insight for her and step by step helped her to appreciate and understand the power of her exclusive personality. She has innate talents other people have to fight for and have to invest energy to become world class.

Her challenge: She could relate to 3 of her 5 top 5 talent themes right from the beginning: Achiever®, Relator® and Adaptability®. But with the other two, Belief® and Ideation®, she needed a bit more time. She did not see the values guiding her in her life (Belief®) and her daily routine offered her little to no time to be creative as often as she wanted and needed it to be (Ideation®). But, isn't it a big success to become aware of these challenges at this point?

Her talents prepared her for her life. In the right environment, she will rise and with the confidence and awareness that these are real talents and not some kind of flaws, Sarah will transform the talents into real strengths. Step by step.

Knowledge and awareness of what she needs to do her best every day is the key to become more of who she really is. And that growing self-confidence will support Sarah to appreciate and understand the unique power of the people around her as well. This will eliminate stress. Sarah will understand that some people just deliver their performances differently than she would do it. Because they are different. Another big point for personal development.

Another important note to highlight at this point is: Each one of your talent themes has many different facets. Embracing your own talent themes is much easier if you know more than just one—keep looking to understand more and more as you develop your talents. As I mentioned before, a talent theme is multi-dimensional and every single time you look at them, you will learn something new! So keep looking and keep in mind, that "every step you take, every move you make" you are supported and guided by your talents.

Sarah's and Your Take Away from E:

Understand your own, personal beauty; what makes you so different. You may be thinking, *There is not a lot I can do, I can't see the value!"*

I will tell you, here is the point:

The main reason we feel stressed is because we have no clue who we are. **E** is the beginning to you being able to fully understand see your beauty and uniqueness. **E** is the beginning to see and appreciate the beauty of the people around you. Build the foundation for your own, personal comfort zone!

You have your top 5 talent themes, which probably seem pretty common to you because they are just that—your talents—and you have always had them. However, others who don't possess these natural gifts, would have to invest a lot of energy and effort into becoming world class in what you see as common.

E of ENJOY will help you with this realization, to embrace the beauty you bring to the world. Simple as that. Understand to LOVE every facet of your talent theme. The more you know and love your talent themes and yourself, the more powerful you are going to be. You are perfect.

Use the reports you got from Gallup and prepare your own questions. Start to create your own, personal comfort zone.

N - Nurture

Stress Occurs When:

1. You are not aware of your talents and thus, do not develop them into strengths that can be used to your advantage.

2. You do not use your talents to their full potential, possibly because you are not completely aware of them.

3. You focus your efforts in areas that conflict with your natural talents, which makes them weaknesses.

In this section, you get to know your talents even better, and expand your comfort zone as much as possible.

Step **N - NURTURE** - of the ENJOY process is mainly designed to help you understand how:

- Each individual talent theme can cause you to feel stressed.
- Each talent theme can help you avoid stress.
- Not using your talent themes at all, not enough, or too much in your daily life with other people could become a huge stressor. Remember, no one is responsible for you stress but YOU!
- Other talent themes in conjunction with your top 5 talent themes can help you be even more effective and confident when facing life's challenges.

Let Me Highlight 2 Things:

1. The fact that talents are neutral takes out any rating or evaluation. Talents explain how you think, act, and feel without any assessment. This is what you need to grow. It expresses the difference of each individual, nothing more and nothing less. You are finally going to be able to explain and show others what things you need in order to work effectively; an incredible opportunity!

2. It will also give you the chance to figure out what went wrong when the result of your actions was not satisfactory. Self-perception and the perception of others are the key concepts here. What is okay for you can be perceived as hurtful or offensive to other people. This gives you the chance to use this

information to reflect on your behavior and then change how you act in the future.

Therefore, you can influence whether you cause new stress and how you deal with existing stress. Like I said, stress develops because you feel powerless. With ENJOY, you are in control! You build up your very own protection mechanisms against stress with your top 5 talent themes. You build up your plan and develop your own strategies for preventing stress.

And, remember: you are in charge of how you act, feel, and behave in different situations. It's all about you. You are not a machine—but are made up of emotions—and they influence your behavior every single day.

N of the ENJOY process will help you become more and more independent from external influence. It's not your coworker or employee who stresses you, it's your limited ability to deal with who you are. **N** will support you to refocus on yourself and help you understand what YOU can do to better deal with stress than you have in the past. You are guided by a combination of talents and like a chef in the kitchen you use different spices to create different dishes.

The combination of your talents, thoughts, and behavior changes depending on each specific situation and on who is around you. With this language, you can better recognize and understand your behavior; and prevent stress. You are the one in charge of protecting and developing yourself. No one else is going to do it for you.

Your goal should be to improve your life and to help you be a valuable member of your community. This helps you to avoid misunderstandings in society, communicate on a whole different level, and ask other people for things they are actually able to accomplish. This creates a different kind of togetherness.

You have to make yourself aware each and every day that you are only human. And humans are not perfect which is okay. It becomes a problem for you and everyone around you when the human element is not further developed. If being human in not further developed, either intentionally or unintentionally, this causes stress—for you and for others.

This is exactly where the **N** in ENJOY comes from.

Effective Stress and Burnout Prevention with Your Own Stress Protection Plan

You deliberately can use your greatest potential, your talents, to protect yourself against stress and burnout. You can use your very own resources. They are the best possible prevention because they have no limits! And you can achieve your goals yourself!

Develop YOUR own personal protection mechanism! After **E** in ENJOY— gaining insights about the own self—you know more of what is special about your talent theme or what you are particularly good at. You started to create YOUR comfort zone.

Now let's move on - to **N** - Nurture your talent themes and develop them to protect you against Stress and Burnout.

I will demonstrate this step explaining how Sarah was introduced to **N** of the ENJOY process. What kind of facts could cause stress for Sarah and how could she use this knowledge to protect herself from it?

Talent Theme: ACHIEVER®

What could cause Sarah stress?	- Constant dissatisfaction, imbalance, and restlessness. - Constantly overlooking your own needs. - "Slackers" - people who don't have the same attitude. - You cannot say no and take on too many tasks.
How can she use the talent theme for protection?	- Learn to say no. - Be mindful of your own needs. - Make plans and lists and stick with them.
How could Sarah complete her mosaic of possibilities?	Having someone to remind her that she has to keep her work ethic in check (maybe someone with Focus®), and connecting with someone strong in relationships building (maybe someone with WOO®) to provide her with social contacts to help get her ideas out and be heard.

Talent Theme: BELIEF®

What could cause Sarah stress?	- Environment where values are not respected. - Unplanned changes in direction dictated from the outside. - Others take advantage of your ethics and selflessness.
How can she use the talent theme for protection?	- Create a list to support your clarity and an overview of your values so you can explain them to yourself and others. - Stubbornness can lead to a lot of resentment against you in others. - Explore other topics to gain flexibility and understanding with a combination of topics.
How could Sarah complete her mosaic of possibilities?	Combining the flexibility provided by her talent theme Adaptability® with this talent theme would be perfect. The train tracks she is living her life on can be so much more effective by using exploring opportunities on being more flexible. Having someone to explain her approach to life would be beneficial, too (maybe someone with Communication®).

Talent Theme: ADAPTABILITY®

What could cause Sarah stress?	- Jobs and projects where this talent is not needed or recognized. - You have no opportunity to react and practice flexibility. - Predefined ways for solving problems.
How can she use the talent theme for protection?	- Seek out flexible people and environments. - Look for jobs where this talent is needed. - Help people in stressful situations.
How could Sarah complete her mosaic of possibilities?	Intentionally using the theme dynamics of her Achiever® and her Adaptability®, on to react more flexibly, the other to finish the new challenge. Someone who could help Sarah focus and concentrate on her goals could be a great addition (maybe someone with Discipline®). In times of stress it could take pressure off her if she could focus on what she is good at and have a person who is focused on the bigger picture (maybe someone with Connectedness®)

Talent Theme: RELATOR®

What could cause Sarah stress?	- When your friendship and trust are taken advantage of. - Cliques. - You have no friends or your group of friends changes frequently. - You have no one-on-one conversations with your colleagues/your boss.
How can she use the talent theme for protection?	- Demonstrate confidence, this will eventually result in a chain reaction. - Do not change your behavior because you were disappointed, but rather learn to use other talents that give you "advance warning" when you are being taken advantage of.
How could Sarah complete her mosaic of possibilities?	This talent theme could use the energy and openness of someone strong in the areas of building multiple relationships (maybe someone with WOO®). Someone outgoing and positive to make connections and prepare the ground for Sarah to be her best self (maybe someone with Includer® or Positivity®).

Talent Theme: IDEATION®

What could cause Sarah stress?	- An inflexible environment, no free space, time pressure. - No opportunities to create and apply ideas. - "The bird must be able to fly, but it can't when it is sitting in a cage"
How can she use the talent theme for protection?	- Create awareness of your talent's needs. Find jobs in which you have freedom. - Schedule time to be able to promote this talent. - Pay attention to time management in order to find a balance between creating too many or not enough ideas.
How could Sarah complete her mosaic of possibilities?	Over and over again—this talent theme needs freedom and the opportunity to be creative. Together with her talent theme of Adaptability®, Ideation® can use the flexibility created by Adaptability® to be more creative. Someone with strong in self-confidence (maybe someone with Self-Assurance®) and with the understanding of what is important to her (maybe someone with Strategic®) would support her to create the environment where she can act and grow. In addition, a creative person like she is, needs optimistic and positive people around them (maybe someone with Positivity®) to help supports her to create ideas from nothing.

The question here is:

How can you use the insights from your dominant talents to prevent stress and burnout?

This is only possible if you have a true understanding of who you are, what your comfort zone is and what could damage your power. You have to be honest about what you can do and what not. It's a learning process. It may take some time, but it is worth it!

ENJOY provides you with the confidence to reflect on your life from a new perspective—understanding who you are!

Sarah's and Your Take Away from N:

Gaining awareness of how your talents can create stress and of how your talents can prevent stress. Gaining awareness of how you think, feel and behave, as well as for your talents, is a big step towards effective stress prevention. But it's just the beginning. We just got started.

Your goal is to create a new plan that replaces the old one, that wasn't working. Let's move on to **J** - Jump - and restructure your life! Create your plan!

J - Jump

Routine and Habits

When you are stressed, you are not able to make meaningful decisions; you have already learned that much. This is why it is important to take precautions which help you to move forward, or at least not move backward when you are in stress mode. These precautions are the so-called routines. They are like stable pillars that do not break down regardless of how stressful the situation. They are what you fall back on when you feel stress coming on, to take the stress off.

If you don't already have a system of routines and habits in place, you will have to jump into new ones. Remember the swimming pool? Picture yourself standing on the edge, preparing to jump in. Ready, set, go - JUMP

An example of this is an impressive story that happened on Tuesday, September 9, 2001. It was the day on which the world seemed to stand still for a moment. It was the day when the two towers of the World Trade Center in New York collapsed after a terrorist attack, and 2,606 people lost their lives.

Rick Rescorla's[13] task was civil protection. After a successful career in the Army, he worked for Morgan Stanley. Morgan Stanley occupied 22 floors in the World Trade Center. He feared that the World Trade Center would be a potential target for terrorists, which is why Morgan Stanley employees did regular evacuation exercises. Rick put in place a routine that everyone could fall back on in an emergency.

When he sent an alarm, everything had to be dropped and orders had to be followed. A team leader was assigned to each floor—and these team leaders had to complete extra training. Their task was to ensure that all employees were able to follow the instructions. Even visitors received a detailed briefing before they could resume their activities.

In other words, the employees established this routine over many years. Again, and again. It became natural for them to know how to react in case of an emergency. They learned to automatically drop everything and to make their lives priority number one.

Then came September 11, 2001—the day that changed a lot of things … and cost a great deal of lives. The first airplane hit tower 1 at 8:46 a.m. The Morgan Stanley offices were located in tower 2. The employees saw what happened and felt the shock.

Rick immediately began to implement the plan that had been practiced for a long time. He ordered his team leaders to start the evacuation immediately. They knew what they were doing, they were trained for it. The plan was executed perfectly; people reacted as soon as they received the order to behave in accordance with the plan. They had been prepared for it for a long time.

---

[13]   https://en.wikipedia.org/wiki/Rick_Rescorla

Exactly 17 minutes later, at 9:03 a.m., the 2nd Airplane hit tower 2. There were shocks, noise and dust, screams, and pure stress. But the people continued to follow the plan they had practiced many years. They did not question anything—they simply followed their routine in spite of the stress and deadly terror that was going on around them. Rick himself, kept control of the situation and made sure that his team continued executing the plan.

By 9:45 a.m., the Morgan Stanley offices were almost completely evacuated. Rick went back one more time because a handful of employees were missing—in addition to some members of his safety team. Everyone knew that Rick would not come out until each and every one of his people was accounted for.

Rick was last seen around 10:00 a.m., in the stairwell of the 10th floor. Sadly, the tower collapsed shortly afterwards. Amazingly, only 13 Morgan Stanley employees died in the terror attack that day. Among them was Rick Rescorla and 4 members of his safety team.

2,687 employees and 250 visitors of Morgan Stanley survived. They survived thanks to Rick Rescorla, the hero, and his foresight. The fact that all employees were used to this routine helped them all to push aside the paralyzing effects of stress. Instead, they were able to save their lives. They survived—because Rick Rescorla had a plan.

What can you learn from this heroic story?

You can prepare for times in which you are exposed to many challenges. The best preparation is to have a plan. A plan that tells you exactly what your routine should look like. A plan that prepares you in case there is stress, it is that simple.

Start and create your OWN plan! A plan created by you, for you, by using your exclusive combination of talents and strengths. And the knowledge about various stress and burnout prevention techniques.

This has been said—you've already started creating YOUR plan. With **E** and **N** of the ENJOY process.

J – Your plan

Let's include in your plan the topic J - JUMP

Imagine, what could be if in any situation—stressful or not—you had a plan you could always count on to make your next important move? What are the most important requirements for such a plan?

It has to be YOUR plan.

But how can it be or become your plan? It has to be grounded on who you are, how you think, and how you behave! It has to be based on what defines your unique way of looking at the world; on what only you can give to make this world a better place!

YOUR TALENTS!

But the talents are just the foundation—they have to be developed into solid strengths. Remember—you develop a talent into a strength by investing time, knowledge and skills. I talked about it in Chapter 2.

E + N of the ENJOY process is the beginning. Now, in **J** you'll make the next big step—you JUMP—because it's a huge and important step. Are you ready? If your answer is "Yes", download the bonus material on my website www.strengths4you.com/bonus-material.

You'll find:

- A "Secret Contract—Decision" and
- A plan—YOUR PLAN.

Part of JUMP is that you decide you are ready to say "Goodbye" to your old behavior and make room for a new way to approach life with a plan—YOUR PLAN—tailored for your needs. This plan will prepare you for any challenge, both in your personal life and in your professional life.

A big plus for your plan is that you will always have the chance to reflect, review, and revise it. Your self-awareness will grow by applying this plan and your knowledge of what you need, what is good for you and who you are, will reach new and unexpected levels.

In order to support your "Goodbye" to the old pattern and behaviors and to prepare the soil for a different future, you are invited to print the "Secret Contract" of the bonus material, read it, adjust it and sign it. www.strengths4you.com/bonus-material.

You need to sign this contract—your brain works in pictures—the signature will help you to hold yourself accountable to continue the new path. After the ink is dry, move on—JUMP and start with your PLAN.

Take the document provided in the bonus material and phrase your GOAL. Create your future, it is your responsibility to yourself. What are you dreaming of? What is the most important dream you want to realize? What is the biggest achievement you can dream of? There is no right and wrong answer here, it's about your hopes and dreams. You have the chance to change your goal at any time ... if you decide that your goal is to have ice cream—it's fine ... next time you can be more courageous and aim for something bigger. ☺

After your goal is defined, you want to start filling in the more detailed parts of your PLAN. The foundation of your future, your plan—everything—is who you are. Your talents! That is area **E**. And again—it's just the beginning. You need to develop your talents into solid strengths. Exactly what are you good at and how can you repeat your success stories over and over again? Add skills and knowledge to them and the investment to understand more and more of the power behind your own self. Fall in love with your talents.

The next area to fill in is **N**. Just use the insights you got from the step **N** of the ENJOY process and fill in the plan. Build on what makes you stand out from others, continue to realize what situations and facts you could create by ignoring your needs and demands. Build awareness of what stresses you and how your talents are there to create stress protection shields.

Done? Okay, great!!! Let's move on!

This plan is supposed to support you to design a new, more efficient and joyful routine to live your life to the fullest. Now, in **J** you will focus on how you can best incite this routine even more. If this support were to come from the outside, you would become dependent and weak—it absolutely has to come from inside of you and, it is possible.

Yes, you are exactly right on it! The support comes from within. You have everything in you to get this done and achieve your boldest goals. It's your body and your mind that are your most important servants! How?

J - Mind / Brain

You are the boss. You are in charge. You are responsible for what you are thinking and where your thoughts are wandering. That needs practice but, it's worth it. Include this intentional practice in your plan. MOVE YOUR BRAIN. Train your mind.

In any stressful situation—and these situations will enter your life as long as you live—you need to have your plan on how to get your mind in a creative, happy, and positive mood. Include in your plan the question:

"Is my life in danger?" Repeat this question 5 times in a row. I can just see you laughing out loud. But, asking yourself this question honestly eliminates the biggest creator of fear: danger—the fear of death. This question will help your brain realize that your life is not threatened by your boss, or your partner. After you have repeated this question 5 times, move your thoughts towards the goal you wrote on top of this document.

CONGRATUALTIONS! You moved your brain. Simple as that. Now, with your focus on what you want and what you are dreaming of, approach your tasks and get them done! ☺

Mindful practice to "move your brain" several times every day, will help you make this a habit and help you refocus. If your thoughts are wandering, wander them towards something else. Practice this habit over and over again—prepare yourself for the future. Wire your brain to become more flexible and adjustable.

Meditation or the usage of Mudra Cards is another way to practice the habit of moving the brain. Make the commitment to yourself that you will dedicate time every single day to practice this point.

We are not done yet! There is one more servant ready to support you on your journey!

J - Body

Your body is your second, most important helper. How?

If you feel stuck, move your body—simple as that. The movement of your body will pull your brain along. Once more, it needs practice. As

Rick Rescorla practiced over and over again to get the staff of Morgan Stanley ready, you need to prepare yourself to be ready in stressful situations. Prepare yourself now! Get started. MOVE YOUR BODY.

One way to do this is just by getting up from your chair and walking around your desk a couple of times. You may even decide to walk your dog, if you have one, even for 5 minutes. Or—my favorite way to move my body is, moving my body to Starbucks and working at one of the tables there. The point is to get yourself out of the immediately, stressful situation if you can.

If it happens for you that you find a bigger slot in your daily routine, include physical exercise in your plan. Maybe you want to sign up for a membership at a local gym or you want to resume your jogging practice. This is the beauty of this plan—you can find your own, unique way to complete it. It's your plan, find what works best for you, even if other people think you're crazy.

It's your life, so get yourself away from the expectations others may have for you, focus on you and YOUR plan. What could work for you? How many minutes of your time daily are you willing to dedicate to this point?

Start slow, and add more minutes when you feel comfortable.

You are on your way, keep going!

Sarah was on her way, too. She got more and more excited and energized with each day. She felt protected by her own self. She realized how this plan supported her to take self-care, so that she could prevent experiencing more stress than necessary.

Her first reaction reading the question "is your life in danger?" got her laughing too, but very soon she felt the true power behind the question—and just smiled big.

Sarah's and Your Take Away From J:

Life is too short to continue a life that makes you sick and sad. Take a chance—and **J** - JUMP—for a better future.

Sarah's plan is progressing. Let's move on to **O** – Optimize and organize.

O - Optimize

A very effective and crucial support to live a self-regulated and healthy life includes a unique, well thought out and optimized organization of 3 important aspects of your life: Sleep, Nutrition and Time. As we continue to design your personal plane, let's start with sleep.

O - Optimized Sleep Routine

Sleep is necessary for stress and burnout prevention. Lack of sleep severely impairs your performance. In the USA, sleep problems cost businesses approximately 411 billion dollars and losing 1.2 million working days a year[14].

Lack of sleep is the reason for high error rates in companies. But sleep problems are also a clear signal your body sends when you are not well. When the mind can no longer be still, thoughts are constantly going through your head. This happens when you no longer have control over your mind—but instead your mind has control over you. Sleep

---

[14] Fortune Health, Lack of Sleep Costs U.S. About $411 Billion, (Nov.2016)

problems are responsible for serious health problems[15] such as heart disease, concentration problems, and even various types of accidents.

Earlier, we were talking about the sympathetic nervous system (SNS) and the parasympathetic nervous system (PNS). The SNS is active when an action is required, as opposed to the PNS, which is active when you are in recovery mode. Here, the organs can relax, the cells can regenerate, and you can recharge your batteries.

The 2 systems should complement each other and create ideal conditions for you to live a healthy and successful life.

Stress has an impact on your nervous system. When you feel stressed, the SNS is at work for the most part. When the SNS is highly active, sleep is often out of the question because when your life is in danger, it could be deadly to fall asleep.

The ENJOY process is your solution for being able to deal with stress and burnout in a healthy way and more effectively, because it includes an optimized approach to sleep. Your new approach is based on what you need and what you learned moving through this process.

High performance athletes place great importance on getting enough sleep. If there is no sleep routine, it is difficult to be resilient and above all, successful in challenging situations. But if there is a sleep routine in place, your body will be prepared to support you as best as possible.

And here is another major advantage: If your body is used to a sleep routine, it is much easier to return to this pattern after challenging situations.

---

[15] Division of Sleep Medicine at Harvard Medical School

This is why I believe it is essential to have a sleep routine optimized for our needs. It must be deliberately incorporated into your overall daily routine, in your plan. Habits are not formed out of the blue. You have to consciously take control to achieve your goals, just like with everything else.

Your Steps to Include Sleep into Your ENJOY Process:

- Be aware of your own sleep habits.
- Plan your daily schedule. Sleep must become firmly established in your plan. Now that you know how important sleep is, make room for it. No one can do this for you! You only have one body to take you on our journey in this world. The better you treat it, the more successful and healthy you will be.
- If you don't have a routine, establish one today.
- Use your new plan to remind you of your best sleeping routine.
- Consciously decide how many hours of sleep you need, and make a note on your plan—hold yourself accountable!

How did we use this for Sarah's exclusive ENJOY plan?

Very simple, she was introduced to the 3 steps I mentioned earlier. Sometimes you can't handle what you are dealing with because you didn't have the idea to think about it. So, it's about awareness. And about acting on the new insights you get out of this process. With Sarah, we included the sleeping routine in her "secret contract." She made the decision to time herself for at least 6-7 hours of sleep every night. She included sleep in her very own ENJOY process.

Remember, you only have this one life ... a slight change of the old routine could make a big difference.

O - Optimized Nutritional Plan

What is the purpose of nutrition? Correct, physical survival. Today it is common knowledge, that nutrition also has an influence on your psyche. There are substances in your food that directly affect the brain.

Professor Emeran Mayer at the University of California, Los Angeles, and one of the leading researchers in the field of neurogastroenterology says, that "Psychiatrists have never before searched for the causes of problems below the neck. In the future, maybe we will treat psychological problems not only in the brain but also in the gastrointestinal tract."[16]

The important thing is **what** and **how** you eat! Because **everything** you eat has an effect. Data analyzed by various research groups showed that people who eat fresh vegetables, fruit, fish, and whole grains have a considerably lower risk of depression. Healthy food will become a great supporter for your brain!

Your intestines and brain are your body's dream team. They are responsible for supplying your body with the right substances at the right time. But since the brain cannot directly absorb the nutrients you need, you've got your intestines for help.

The intestines and the brain are connected to each other through the vagus nerve, which transmits signals in both directions—but 90% of these signals are transmitted from the gastrointestinal tract to the brain! This is why it is so important to incorporate the intestines in stress prevention.

---

[16]   Mayer,E.A. (2016) .The Mind Gut Connection. New York. Harper Wave.

Prerequisites for Optimum Function of our Intestines:

- Enough good quality oxygen
- Enough sleep
- Enough exercise
- Adequate rest
- A lot of fluids
- Energy in the form of food
- Eating in line with our circadian rhythm

All of this is very important but, nutrition is the most important point. Healthy nutrition cannot be replaced by sleep, oxygen, or exercise. It can only be supplemented. The gut is not an **individual player**, but is a part of the "dream team" in conjunction with the brain.

Without question, the gut is much more than a digestive organ. In the intestines, your metabolism is controlled in close cooperation with the brain.

You might not fully understand the importance of the metabolic processes in the intestines. Perhaps you don't even want to fully understand it. The visible end product of the intestinal function may be the main reason for many people not to want to understand this process.

The intestines are responsible for your wellbeing and for ensuring that all organs work properly. Disturbing the metabolic process not only disrupts the growth and generation processes in the body, but also the function of your immune system and your overall health.

As complex and remarkable as the metabolic process may be, contrary to popular belief: you need a surprisingly small amount of nutritional elements in the form of solid food: carbohydrates, fats, proteins, vitamins, and minerals. In other words, your ancestors' diet was actually pretty good. And what about today?

Nutrition plays an important role in preventing the diseases and problems you face today. This is especially true when it comes to stress.

Nutrition Influences How You Deal with Stress

Nutrient deficiency can develop when either not enough nutrients are produced or when too many nutrients are broken down due to certain conditions (such as stress) and are no longer available to the body. The efficiency of the brain depends on whether there is a lack of micro or macro nutrients or a combination thereof or a lack of adequate concentrations of supplements. If neurotransmitters crucial for nerve function are missing, brain power will be limited. The susceptibility for stress does not increase solely due to life events, but also when you don't provide your brain with the nutrients it needs.

How Can You Help Boost Your Performance Level?

Fluid—Water

An adult's body is up to 60% water; a child's body might even consist of up to 75%. Water is not food but it is necessary for all metabolic functions in the body: Building of cells, digestion, cardiovascular circulation, and heat regulation. It helps detox the body through the kidneys and the liver. It supports the immune system by keeping the mucous membranes moist, and thins the blood to ensure that oxygen in transported through the body.

Humans can survive without solid food for some time—but only a few days without water. In other words, supplying the body with an adequate amount of water is vital to survival.

Protein/Amino Acids

Amino acids and proteins provide valuable basic elements for the production of skin, hair, muscles, hormones, enzymes, and cells. And as I said, amino acids play an important role in terms of brain function. Since only a very limited amount of proteins can be stored in the body, they have to be consumed regularly.

Fatty Acids

Saturated and unsaturated fatty acids are very important for the development and function of the nerve membranes. Fatty acids typically lack a sufficient amount of unsaturated Omega-3 fatty acids. However, they are extremely important for effective brain function.

In countries such as Japan where people eat a lot of fish, depression is much rarer. The explanation may lie in Omega-3 fatty acids which the body cannot produce on its own. Omega-3 fatty acids can be found in algae, plants, or fish in the form of ester.

Vitamins and Minerals

There is probably not a single vitamin or mineral that does not affect our brain one way or another. They are necessary, among other things, for the development of neurotransmitters and fatty acids. Without them, synthesis would not be able to take place. They are also necessary for energy production.

If there is a lack of vitamins or minerals, the concentration of neurotransmitters and fatty acids decreases and brain function is severely restricted. Group B vitamins play a vital role here. All of them are water-soluble and can be mainly found in meat and whole grains. Because they are water-soluble, they don't have a very long shelf life and loose essential vitamins after a short period of time.

Through your nutrition, you have the opportunity to impact your susceptibility to stress!

This is an important point Sarah was more than astonished about. After realizing how easy she could support her body to sustain stress on a different level, she included this topic in her plan. The ENJOY process was a great reminder for her. Sarah took notes that she wanted to invest time to set up a nutrition plan. She embraced her responsibility to do this.

Again, sometimes it's enough to create awareness. If you know why you should do something, it can be pretty easy to change an old behavior.

O - Optimized Time Management

Time management is another important aspect of your plan, and more and more than anything else, it has to be set up how your brain needs it. Time management is kind of like the curb on your street to success. It guides you in situations where you might have lost the perspective.

Setting up a time management pattern helps guide you back to what you want, and how you can get there when things get stressful or difficult. It is important to organize your time the way you need it. The best way to do this is to use the unique combination of your Clifton Strengths® talent themes.

Our talents determine how we see the world. This includes how we manage our time. Successful time management means you have to know your own limits and to be able to set realistic goals. To be able to use the time you have available in the most efficient way possible.

Time management is not just an integral part of successful stress prevention; it is vital. But, only if you understand how to tailor it to your own individual needs. Time management is an outstanding example how you can use the Clifton Strengths® to reach your goals when you know the facets of your own talents inside and out. **Aim your talents to set up a time management that works for you! Optimize your routines.**

The question you have to ask yourself is, "How can I use my talent themes to complete my tasks as efficiently and fully as possible."

Start by defining your goal then take the definitions of your top 5 Clifton Strengths® talent themes. Read through them carefully. Highlight words and phrases that will answer this question: "How can this talent theme support me to achieve my goal of effective time management?"

It may be the fact that Analytical® could help you "analyze the given facts" or Focus® could help with the "perseverance to continue until the goal is achieved."

Over the years, I have found the following exercise to me very effective: take your Clifton Strengths® Discovery Cards / Clifton Strengths® Theme Insights Cards and put the ones that match your top 5 talent themes in front of you on the table. How can each talent theme give you an answer? Trust me, each talent theme provides you with a facet that can help you achieve your goals. Your joy is in finding the facets within each talent theme.

This task offered lots of fun for Sarah. Guess which talent theme was more than happy to be used? Correct—Ideation®—to create a schedule. But Achiever® was a "go to" talent as well. This talent theme includes achieving goals and reaching the finish line. Sarah came up with great ideas on how to organize her days differently, how to best get them started and how to manage her "free time" more effectively.

Including the Relator® in her daily routines showed up in more "one on one" meetings with her employees. She also focused on setting aside specific time for these meetings, to focus on each individual and their needs–instead of wasting time in meetings with everyone.

Adaptability® became her secret weapon! She learned just how to use it and if anything went differently than she had planned, this talent theme would become her flexible advisor on just how to move on.

Each one of her talents had an aspect to support her time management plan. A plan she felt very comfortable and very calm with.

Sarah has a great combination of talents—as you have your great combination as well. All you need is to start using it—in every aspect of your life!

O - Optimize your sleep, nutrition and time. Prepare yourself and get ready!

Sarah's and Your Take Away from O:

It makes absolutely no sense to use a generic development plan. It has to be tailored to your needs. **O** will support you to optimize your plan according to your needs.

Now, let's finish with the cherry on the ice cream: The **Y**—my favorite one. Because all is about **Y** - YOU!

Y - YOU

Everything starts with YOU - and everything ends with YOU. YOU are in charge!

From the time you are born, you are already equipped with pattern. Pattern, more or less flexible. Then you get older, you acquire knowledge that adds to the preexisting pattern. Either at school or after you have earned your degree, you continue to learn.

With ENJOY you have the opportunity to develop the real YOU from the natural patters. To become and to show who YOU are. To let go of old patterns and to develop and showcase the uniqueness of your own personality.

Yes - it is up to YOU to become YOU. To do this, you need knowledge and courage. New wisdom and new insights. New, because nobody like you has ever lived before. There is no information available on what YOU have to do to be happy and successful. Allow yourself the freedom and the courage to acquire this knowledge. This applies to all aspects of your life. To all issues you may face. You are free! You set your own limits. Nobody else. To free you from unnecessary stress you have to embrace the whole beauty of yourself - in every aspect of your life. You have to set yourself free before anything else.

How can you inspire yourself to consciously create your own new knowledge base? It is all about YOU, who you are, and what make you unique. YOU are in the spotlight of your knowledge base. This YOU consists of your Clifton Strengths® top 5 talent themes developed into powerful, solid strengths. Your personal plan with several techniques that will help you be the most effective and confident you can possibly be. With behavior that fills your new life with what makes you happiest—relationships, thoughts and activities.

Your unique ENJOY process won't be complete without **Y**. The **Y** starts with two more techniques to set you up for success. Mindfulness und Effective breathing techniques.

Y - Mindfulness - Meditation - YOGA

How does mindfulness benefit personal development and stress and burnout prevention?

John Kabat Zinn[17] is one the most important names when it comes to mindfulness.

What is mindfulness? According to Wikipedia, mindfulness is the psychological process of bringing one's attention to the internal and external experiences occurring in the present moment.

Walk - while you are walking

Look - while you are looking

Listen - while you are listening

Feel - who you really are - now[18]

Mindfulness training is a particularly effective way to learn to be aware of your feelings and behaviors. The goal is to live in the present. In the here and now. To not simply follow others. A certain type of stillness perhaps. Or simply taking a step back. It is a way to direct the focus from the outside to the inside. Regardless of what you do - when you train mindfulness, it is easier for you to live in the present moment. To not only aimlessly live in the future by having plans, goals, and desires.

---

[17] Kabat-Zinn, Jon. (2013). Full catastrophe living : using the wisdom of your body and mind to face stress, pain, and illness. New York :Bantam Books trade paperback.
[18] Nicole Seichter, 2017

Mindfulness is an absolute MUST for stress prevention. If you are not aware of who you are, how you are feeling, and let yourself get swept away in the flurry of events, then your life is all about others - not about yourself.

However, with mindfulness, you can become aware of your own talents and strengths and leverage them. You intentionally redirect your focus from outwards to inwards.

Mindfulness is the opposite of multitasking. You deliberately focus on one task - to become calm and do nothing for example. Through mindfulness, you can learn to become aware of yourself and your actions. When you are in the present moment, you are able to feel and notice what is happening with you right now. The question is whether you have control over your life, whether you can decide yourself, or whether others are deciding for you.

But this does not happen overnight. Be patient with yourself! Get started and include mindfulness in your own ENJOY process. In your plan. I included a couple exercises in my bonus material. Sign up and get started.

Beside practicing mindfulness, you should get used to meditation, too. Meditation is a very effective practice to become more intentional about yourself. Maybe you could add every day 5 minutes of meditation to your daily routine. Meditation is a great way to say intentionally STOP to the craziness of our daily routine. Again—it's about you—you have to make the decision to dedicate time to yourself. You could use this time for a short bible study, for a prayer, or just to breathe. And doing nothing else.

Besides this, YOGA would be a great help for you to become more intentional. And, don't get scared. YOGA is not just meant to be for young flexible people. Everywhere studios are offering different styles and levels of Yoga. It's you—again—who decides what is good for you and what is just too much. You have just one vehicle on this planet—your body—treat it wisely! No one else will do this for you!

Sarah included this point **Y** in her "contract with herself" and in her plan to optimize her life. Each day one technique to practice mindfulness or a short meditation followed her along. In the beginning, she needed the plan to remind her - but more and more it became a habit.

Y - Develop Conscious Breathing Patterns

I cannot stress often enough how important breathing is. Life starts with an inhale - and ends with an exhale. This is how it has been since the beginning of time - and always will be. This is reason enough to raise awareness about the breath and include it in any program to prevent stress and burnout.

"The universal life force is enhanced and guided through the harmonious rhythm of the breath."[19]

"Our breath is the bridge from our body to our mind, the element which reconciles our body and mind and which makes possible oneness of body and mind. Breath is aligned to both body and mind and it alone is the tool which can bring them both together, illuminating both and bringing both peace and calm."[20]

---

[19] Nuernberger, P. (1978). The quest for personal power.
[20] Nhất Hạnh, Thích. (1987). The miracle of mindfulness : a manual on meditation. Boston :Beacon Press.

Over the years, you forget how important breathing is for your wellbeing. Being aware of what breathing means to you and, above all, how important it is in helping with your daily challenges is often blurred by things that are supposedly more important.

What can be more important than breathing? You can go for weeks without eating. You can also manage without fluids for a few days. But when you don't breathe, it has instant consequences. This includes cognitive consequences, physical impairments - and even death. Your breath is the most important source of energy for the body. The breath combines the systems of your body.

Breath is an important anchor in stress and burnout prevention because while it provides you with energy, your breath helps with the process of developing the YOU. Letting go of habits and developing your own YOU will be enforced by an effective technique to breathe.

This most effective, of course, if you have first expanded your own unique comfort zone applying **E, N, J** and **O** as much as possible with the help of your talents. After this, conscious and trained breathing provides major support with personal development. This is why it is such a vital part of ENJOY and why a conscious breathing pattern should be part of your ENJOY process. Include it in your new routine, your plan.

The main purpose of breathing is to supply our blood with oxygen - which filters toxic substances out of our body. But this is not all—through the breath, you can take control of your body and, above all, consciously manage stress. The connection between breathing and the autonomic nervous system is behind this. Through this connection, you control the amount of oxygen in your body as well as the emotional reactions of your body. This permits a healthier and more self-determined life.

ENJOY is a holistic and well thought through process. A process that celebrates the unique power each one of us can offer. For the benefit of ourselves and others!

Y – The Final Touch

You take your car to the car wash pretty regularly, right? After the car has been cleaned, there is a usually a "final rinse". This last step is a simple procedure to make the clean car shine even more. It not only helps make the car shine that much brighter, it makes it even more visible to everyone that your car just got cleaned. ☺

The final touch or "final rinse" in this case is the procedure to sharpen the edges of your ENJOY process, wrap up your vigorous approach and turn it back towards the outside. **Y** is the act of getting your plan from the ME to the WE. This is the way we have a true impact on our lives.; your opportunity to change the world—one step at a time.

You want to know how?

After building the intense and powerful self-awareness, while creating your plan, implement the ENJOY process to every area of your life! Yes, correct. Every area of your life, both inside and out.

ENJOY has helped you to better understand who you are, and has opened your eyes to what you need in order to avoid unnecessary stress. You have created a realistically new routine to approach life. And ENJOY has guided you to optimize your life exactly how you need it. Now it's time to aim all of this towards the outside—towards the people you love, the people you work with and the others you come in contact with every day.

Every breath you take, every move you make, your Clifton Strengths® top 5 are always with you. Use this new self-awareness and dive into every part and facet of the YOU. Become as confident as you can. Become courageous. Become demanding. Become YOU!

Fill your mind, spirit and soul only with what you deserve. Use what you have learned about yourself from Clifton Strengths® to examine the world around you. And, it's again about asking questions:

- What and who fills your buckets. Lovingly observe and question yourself and others.

- Did you set boundaries? Who and what inspires you to do what you do? Is there anything that drains you but you don't know how to stop it?

- Did you find words and phrases to explain your new level of self-awareness to others? Don't expect them to know about the changes you are making, you have to tell them.

- Take your secret contract and reflect on it—anything to add? Something you want to remove?

- Reflect on your plan, over and over again—anything you like to add? Anything you'd like to remove?

This final touch, the spirited self-examination and the changes you'll make, will permit you to be the most authentic you. The butterfly effect will be seen and experienced by you, and those around you. You know what you deserve and you will claim it.

You will become a role model for others and you will see that you have started to change the world! One day at a time—one person at a time.

Just get started! Believe in who you are and the things that only you can give to this world—your true self.

ENJOY guided Sarah towards becoming super extraordinary! Self-awareness is fueled by permanent reconfirmation of doing the right thing. Including Clifton Strengths® is such an important start to becoming super aware of yourself. In combination with the ENJOY process, a new life is truly possible.

You will finally understand so many things about yourself you somehow practiced before. And with the knowledge that this is now a part of who you are, you are finally able to guide yourself towards a new level of excellence. The same happened with Sarah. She got a powerful self-confidence that showed itself in her being more successful in her professional life AND her personal life. Sarah excitedly moved from feeling weak and stressed, to powerful and ready to accomplish her goals in life.

It's pointless to repeat that effective stress and burnout prevention simply makes sense—if you first create your comfort zone and build on your talent themes. Start with **E** and **N** of the ENJOY process, before you move on! Complete your plan by defining your **J**, **O**, and **Y**.

Sarah joyfully completed her plan by filling topic **Y** with ideas.

Sarah's and Your Take Away from Y:

You have everything inside you to be successful, happy and to find the place you belong. And it's up to YOU to claim this place—don't accept anything else!

I know these all seems like a lot. Just be aware—Rome was not built in one day. Don't stress yourself. It won't happen overnight. The most important thing is to focus on your long-term goal of effective stress prevention for your whole body. And just as when you were learning to drive a car, you may feel very overwhelmed in the beginning by the many different things you have to learn in order to arrive home safe and sound. But step by step, and with a little patience, everything becomes second nature to you. Just get started and be consistent—you will be fine!

CHAPTER 9

Reality Check III

When you use the perspective of Clifton Strengths® in your reality check to look for the causes of stress and burnout in the participants, you will likely find a lot of things that could have been done differently to prevent burnout.

Since it is not possible to make a comparison, I want to illustrate based on their top 5 what (in the affected person's own words) was not observed, and what is different now since they have started observing these things in their daily lives. Working with Clifton Strengths® helped each one of them to become more aware of who they are, and what will help them to prepare for a better future.

Paula

TOP 5	TALENT THEME	WHAT IS SPECIAL ABOUT THIS TALENT?
1	Ideation®	People exceptionally talented in the Ideation® theme are fascinated by ideas. They are able to find connection between seemingly disparate phenomena.
2	Activator®	People exceptionally talented in the Activator® theme can make things happen by turning thoughts into action. They are often impatient.
3	WOO®	People exceptionally talented in the Woo® theme love the challenge of meeting new people and winning them over. They derive satisfaction from breaking the ice and making a connection with someone.
4	Communication®	People exceptionally talented in the Communication® theme generally find it easy to put their thoughts into words. They are good conversationalists and presenters.
5	Empathy®	People exceptionally talented in the Empathy® theme can sense other people's feelings by imagining themselves in others' lives and situations.

What Could Have Been Different?

You cannot change the past, you can only analyze it to see what was missing, and what could have been done differently to produce a more favorable outcome. Which strengths were not used to their potential, or which strengths were used too much and caused the body to feel it had no other way out than to switch to emergency mode—burnout?

An important issue for Paula was that because of the reorganization and getting a new boss, she was no longer able to use her strengths of Activator® or Ideation®. When she first started working at the company, she had the opportunity to use these strengths and was very happy, fulfilled, and successful.

Her Communication® and Woo® skills also worked in her favor. She was respected, completed her projects with enthusiasm and commitment, had space and opportunities to be creative, and implemented the ideas she had.

The approach of her new supervisor is what got her troubles started. Suddenly, all of her creativity was eliminated, and she no longer had the ability to initiate new projects. Therefore, Paula no longer had the opportunity to interact with clients and customers.

A change within the company was also without success—she was simply unable to express what she needed to be effective. The system in her organization was not flexible enough to match her uniqueness to a job in which Paula could use her talents. The procedures in the organization did not have any provisions to take this into account. The focus was, and probably still is on the tasks that have to be completed, regardless of who did them. Nobody ever thought about how each employee—or especially Paula—could best be put to use. Her batteries were slowly starting to drain and burnout was the result …

How Did ENJOY Support Her?

ENJOY is a process created to prevent stress and burnout.

Paula started with me after she had her burnout. She wanted to use the ENJOY process to help her understand exactly what happened and how she could avoid the same thing happening again in the future.

She clearly recognized that the work environment, specifically the process within the organization, had been suffocating her. She missed setting boundaries. Step by step, every source of energy had been taken away from her.

After gaining these insights, Paula started to research the facets of her talents in detail and to embrace them wholeheartedly. She also started to learn which alarm signals she can recognize that point to stress within her talents. And she thought about how she could use her unique combination of talents in the future to prevent this from happening again.

Combined with the stress and burnout prevention techniques of ENJOY her solid comfort zone helped her to be prepared for future challenges.

Paula wanted to become a better version of herself—and she continues to use the ENJOY process and the results Clifton Strengths® offers.

Adam

TOP 5	TALENT THEME	WHAT IS SPECIAL ABOUT THIS TALENT?
1	Maximizer®	People exceptionally talented in the Maximizer® theme focus on strengths as a way to stimulate personal growth and group excellence. They seek to transform something strong into something superb.
2	Focus®	People exceptionally talented in the Focus® theme can take a direction, follow through, and make the corrections necessary to stay on track. They prioritize, then act.

TOP 5	TALENT THEME	WHAT IS SPECIAL ABOUT THIS TALENT?
3	Intellection®	People exceptionally talented in the Intellection® theme are characterized by their intellectual activity. They are introspective and appreciate intellectual discussions.
4	Input®	People exceptionally talented in the Input® theme have a craving to know more. Often they like to collect and archive all kinds of information.
5	Futuristic®	People exceptionally talented in the Futuristic® theme are inspired by the future and what could be. They energize others with their visions of the future.

What Could Have Been Different?

As with Paula, we also cannot change Adam's past. We can only analyze it to see what was missing. Which strengths he was not able to use or which strengths were used too much so that the body saw no other way out than to switch to emergency mode—burnout?

In Adam's opinion, the most important point was that he had no control of his own future. He was treated like a number that had to execute commands. Maximizer®, one of his talents, was no longer possible at all. The stored information he had because of his strength Input®, were neither needed or valued by his superiors. And what else should he focus on? Everything was just so pointless. But, he wanted so much more for himself and started to think and think ... and did not want to stop ... until Adam could no longer go on. He was burned out.

How Did ENJOY Support Him?

Adam started the ENJOY process after his burnout as well. He wanted to understand more about WHY things happened the way they did, and he saw the ENJOY process as his tool to help him.

With the ENJOY process, Adam explored how his talents could be used to support him on his way to create something more fulfilling. He understood that, in the long-term, his life could not be centered around a company where he had no chance to create the future or create excellence, for himself or others. Adam got much more confident setting boundaries for himself.

Adam also understood that he had to intentionally invest in his talents on a daily basis to better understand himself. He also learned how to protect himself better against stress. His biggest aha moment came for him during the J of the ENJOY process—the decision to stop repeating old patterns simply because he was used to them. Instead he replaced these old pattern with techniques to support his success and health. Finally he had a plan—his ENJOY plan.

Isabelle

TOP 5	TALENT THEME	WHAT IS SPECIAL ABOUT THIS TALENT?
1	Learner®	People exceptionally talented in the Learner® theme have a great desire to learn and want to continuously improve. The process of learning, rather than the outcome, excites them.
2	Connectedness®	People exceptionally talented in the Connectedness® theme have faith in the links among all things. They believe there are few coincidences and that almost every event has a meaning.

TOP 5	TALENT THEME	WHAT IS SPECIAL ABOUT THIS TALENT?
3	Input®	People exceptionally talented in the Input® theme have a craving to know more. Often they like to collect and archive all kinds of information.
4	Empathy®	People exceptionally talented in the Empathy® theme can sense other people's feelings by imagining themselves in others' lives and situations.
5	Intellection®	People exceptionally talented in the Intellection® theme are characterized by their intellectual activity. They are introspective and appreciate intellectual discussions.

What Could Have Been Different?

Since we cannot change Isabelle's past either, we can only analyze it to see what was missing. Which strengths she could not use or which strengths were used too much so that the body saw no other way out than to switch to emergency mode—burnout?

In Isabelle's opinion, the most important point was that she was not connected at all with her strengths. She did not acknowledge her strengths as such, but rather thought they were commonplace, things that others also possessed. She did not see her uniqueness at all. Instead, she tried to fit into a mold she was pressed into, either intentionally or unintentionally, by others. Until Isabelle could not go on any longer! She was burned out.

How Did ENJOY Support Her?

For Isabelle, the ENJOY process became a tool to prevent her crossing another red light. Through ENJOY, she learned to actually acknowledge her strengths as such. She fell in love with herself, respected herself more and implemented techniques to set herself up for growth.

Today, she no longer tries to develop strengths that are not "right" for her (being more disciplined, being more accurate, etc.), but has lots of fun working with what she has! The plan she created after completing the ENJOY process is her strong "cheat sheet". In uncertain moments this plan is always a great way to get her back on track.

James

TOP 5	TALENT THEME	WHAT IS SPECIAL ABOUT THIS TALENT?
1	Empathy®	People exceptionally talented in the Empathy® theme can sense other people's feelings by imagining themselves in others' lives and situations.
2	Analytical®	People exceptionally talented in the Analytical® theme search for reasons and causes. They have the ability to think about all the factors that might affect a situation.
3	Individualization®	People exceptionally talented in the Individualization® theme are intrigued with the unique qualities of each person. They have a gift for figuring out how different people can work together productively.
4	Relator®	People exceptionally talented in the Relator® theme enjoy close relationships with others. They find deep satisfaction in working hard with friends to achieve a goal.

TOP 5	TALENT THEME	WHAT IS SPECIAL ABOUT THIS TALENT?
5	Maximizer®	People exceptionally talented in the Maximizer® theme focus on strengths as a way to stimulate personal growth and group excellence. They seek to transform something strong into something superb.

What Could Have Been Different?

Again, we cannot change the past, we can only analyze it to see what James was missing. Which strengths he was not able to use or which strengths were used too much so that the body saw no other way out than to switch to emergency mode—burnout?

In James' opinion, the most important issue for him was that there was no appreciation or simply time for what he was doing and for who he was. His Empathy® had to be hidden behind a thick wall which his Maximizer® theme was unable to shine through. Nobody was truly interested in being a team. There was a suicide and several burnouts in the company. He simply did not feel appreciated. He was not able to utilize and further develop his skills.

James could not go on any longer! He was burned out.

How Did ENJOY Support Him?

James started with the ENJOY process to create his unique stress prevention plan to prevent what happened to him before. A plan built just for him. After he realized how important and powerful his talent Empathy® was for himself and his life up to this point, and after he also understood the dynamic of all of the talent themes, he ended up with a completely new perspective. Both for his personal life as well as his career.

He changed his priorities because he realized that he had little chance to use his talents at his current employer or to be assigned jobs or tasks that corresponded to his talents. His most important step: he filled out his first job application in over 20 years, and it was geared towards his talents.

He also started to find out what could cause stress for his talents and developed his own defense mechanisms. The measures to prevent stress and burnout which did very little in the past to help him suddenly had a completely new level of effectiveness. Meditation, breathing exercises, time management all of a sudden made sense.

James finally had his life in his own hands, suddenly felt empowered, and was happier and more satisfied, which his family noticed as well.

Again, ENJOY is a process to prevent stress and burnout. It is not meant to replace a therapy. You can add ENJOY as a tool to help yourself move on but never ignore the help of therapy if you need it. You may complete your treatment with your doctor and start with ENJOY after you are back to a normal life. Talk to your doctor if you are not sure how to act. Remember, you just have this one life to live, be sensitive to your needs.

CHAPTER 10

ENJOY in Your Office

The ENJOY process is your guide for expanding your comfort zone by being aware of and utilizing your talent themes and then employing effective stress and burnout prevention measures. This is very easy in the comfort of our own home.

This new type of communication is your future. You can finally celebrate and benefit from your uniqueness, and even use it to your advantage. However, it would be a waste to use this knowledge only in your personal life. It is also necessary to place the importance you deserve where you spend most of your time—at work! Get started and multiply the power of Clifton Strengths® and the ENJOY process.

When every single person within an organization becomes aware of their own uniqueness, and when it is appreciated and utilized, anything is possible. You enjoy going to work when you know that what you do is important and contributes to the company's success. You are more motivated, healthier, and more prepared to fight not only for yourself but, for your team. The "I" becomes "US"; everybody wins. Here we can find the real power of the ENJOY process! Everything is possible—nothing is impossible!

As a manager or employer the ENJOY process will be your tool to not just use Clifton Strengths® to change the way how to communicate. ENJOY will change the way how you communicate AND change the company culture by creating individual personal development plans for each and every employee.

Managers will become role models because they are part of the team, not just because they are the boss. This helps to recognize the overall performance of the individual parts of the team, and you no longer feel you have to put others down to highlight your own performance. You can find statistics on the Gallup website that confirm this. Employee engagement increases significantly. Employees begin to feel that their impact contributes to the overall goals of the company which has a direct effect on the success of the company itself—both in numbers and in the type of corporate culture that develops.

This is why ENJOY is designed for the individual, but also the entrepreneur, coach and boss. You have the chance and responsibility to grow, for your business—but above all for your employees!

Make sure that your employees can utilize their uniqueness for the benefit of the company and that you go down a new, more successful path towards stress and burnout prevention with my ENJOY process. You will create a considerably more motivating corporate culture, and save millions in the process!

As manager, you should make sure that your competitiveness does not depend solely on whether or not you have enough staff to face challenges, but rather on how your employees can be utilized to keep you one step ahead of the competition. Your employees, customers, and suppliers will undoubtedly help and support you on this course.

Components of ENJOY That Integrate into the Office:

- Clifton Strengths® - General introduction
- **E** for ENJOY
- Clifton Strengths® What, Why, Definitions, Basics - Knowledge of Stress and Burnout
- **N** - in ENJOY - with exercises
- **J** - in ENJOY - with exercises
- **O** - in ENJOY - with exercises
- **Y** - in ENJOY - with exercises

The ultimate goal is to create a work environment in which the unique contribution of each employee can be developed and expanded as much as possible. Using Clifton Strengths® and developing a training plan for each and every employee at the same time.

The ENJOY process is your tool! How can you create a work environment that makes people stay and feel proud to spend their time with you? Employee retention and engagement will increase significantly and happy faces in the hallways and reduced costs will be the side effects of our collaboration.

The goal is for my client's employees to recognize their talents using the ENJOY process and to be able to use them for both personal benefits as well as to benefit their employer. Once this is achieved, they all will have expanded their comfort zone, become familiar with how to use their talents in the most effective ways, and be able to work from a position of strength.

This is the basis for a stress-free work environment. When there are challenges, everyone will know how to deal with them.

A completely new conversation between everybody will start. A conversation of appreciation for, and in recognition of, the uniqueness of each and every person. This provides the opportunity to make everyone's role within the company very clear. But also gives each individual the space to decide HOW to fulfill their role. The leeway that this creates will lead to greater employee loyalty because all employees know that the company believes in their abilities. They will feel appreciated and go to greater lengths to do excellent work.

This will start a cycle that can only be beneficial to all parties involved. ENJOY provides the unique opportunity to approach any challenge with the question: "How can we combine the talents from all of us to get things done." "You don't have to be well rounded—but the team has to be well rounded."

The ENJOY process not ONLY includes Clifton Strengths®, it is a multi-faceted combination of Clifton Strengths® and a wide variety of insights and techniques for stress and burnout prevention. Techniques alone are not enough, our brains need to understand the benefits of learning these techniques. Only then will the highest possible efficiency be guaranteed.

Personal responsibility and motivation are very important aspects for me. I hope to inspire each and every one of my clients to continue with the ENJOY process after the workshop. Independently, or with my support for regular follow-up meetings. Whatever your individual needs may be, I can meet them!

Use my knowledge as a Gallup-Certified Strengths Coach, a certified Stress and Burnout Prevention Coach and use insights from my time as a Yoga instructor to be prepared for the challenges of the future.

Why do you need ENJOY?

To Improve Your System

Your company may be a well-oiled system. Everything seems to be fine. There are ups and downs you have to adjust here and there but, overall you are pleased with the behavior of your employees, your teams and management team; your ROI is increasing every year. But ...

Yes but, yes there is a but. It could be better—employee engagement seems to be down a bit and of course, some of your good employees left recently, and took with them the knowledge and background they got from you over the years. Each one of these great people added a lot of value to the team, and it took you a while to find a replacement for them. In some cases, you had to transfer the new hired staff members to different places, where they fit in better or, in the worst case, terminate their employment.

With ENJOY we will start having a conversation about opportunities to create a new awareness for the employees itself and a new awareness between the management and the employees. Understanding the present situation and creating the picture "what could be".

To improve the system, you have to start with the individual. ENJOY starts with the individual—and with the organization at the same time. Let's get started.

To Prepare for Change

Your company has been developing and growing a lot lately. Your focus has been the growth of the business and now you've come to realize that the old system needs to be restructured! You are likely aware that if you want your business to continue to grow, there must be a change.

Implementing the ENJOY process and realizing the unique impact that each of your employees and coworkers could bring to the table will help give you the leverage you need to continue to grow.

Make everyone understand the need of change and how this will be an advantage for each employee and of course, for the whole management team.

ENJOY is a very inspiring and convincing way to create the soil for change. It's not just about yourself—everyone needs to be on the same path. Everybody is in charge to carry parts of the responsibility. Prepare yourself, the staff and the system for the change and benefit from the fact that the awareness of being a responsible part empowers everybody to contribute so much more to the goal you want to achieve.

To Recreate the System Within Your Business

Your business has been going through a rough time lately. There are red flags all over the place. The old system you used for success did not work. Maybe there are people within your organization creating tension. A high turnover is a clear sign of that. But it just doesn't make sense to fix things just in some areas, you need to recreate a new system and an entirely new company culture. Why not include the ENJOY process to help get you back on the right path?

The ENJOY process will help you understand what exactly needs to be changed in your environment to help each and every team member to be their best! Since it includes the individual development, your toxic environment will be cleaned up, simply because of a higher awareness and knowledge of each person's unique perspective and talents. Because of the improved eagerness to win as a team, a new company culture will be a strong factor to prepare for a successful future.

PARAGON

Paragon Laboratories is a mid-sized company in Michigan. Paragon is one of my clients where I recently had the opportunity to introduce the ENJOY process.

John Parmentier, the president of Paragon, has always been personally fascinated by Clifton Strengths®. One of his top 5 talent themes is Futuristic®. His Futuristic®, as well as the fact that it is always difficult to find qualified and good employees who can be trained for management jobs in the company, prompted Parmentier to develop the "John Spurr School" program in 2015. The program was developed to satisfy Paragon's demand for managers and leadership personalities, which were needed due to the growth of the company as well as the future retirement of present managers.

Parmentier used his talent theme Futuristic® to devise his corporate strategy. *What could be different tomorrow? How can a company's focus be changed to have an advantage over the competition?* The status quo was questioned, which opened new opportunities for a more successful future for the company.

The "John Spurr School" program helps to:

- Find out which employees are interested in management roles.

- Test employees to see whether they are suited for the program.

- Acquire skills and insights into their future roles.

- Enable the company to train employees who can fill the job openings when needed.

- Provide excellent training to the employees, enabling them to manage the company when the free market does not have any qualified employees.

Parmentier recognized that ENJOY would give his program an additional invaluable benefit and hired me. The core values of the company, the vision, and ENJOY were a perfect match.

My ENJOY process was integrated as an additional module into the John Spurr School. I am currently supporting the Alpha group that started in 2015 and will continue until 2018 as well as the Beta group that started in 2016 and will probably be finished in 2019, with one-day to two-day workshops.

Paragon's president is convinced that managers must know their own comfort zone to have control over their own stress level. Once they know their own strengths and weaknesses, they will be able to treat their employees in a completely new way. This allows them to build an effective and trusting partnership with the employees and colleagues—and not only will the employees experience a better work climate, but the customers and suppliers as well.

CHAPTER 11

Rephrase Your Life

Limits

Now that you have arrived at the end of this book, let's address the critics and skeptics. They have always existed in the past and will always exist in the future. This is something we simply have to deal with. This book certainly does not claim to be a universal miracle cure. But, it is a start for people to structure their lives differently and finally have a chance of not wasting another single day being controlled by expectations of others, upbringing, and constraints. Letting go of patterns and developing your OWN YOU.

The ENJOY process will not work if you don't fully believe in your talents. It is certainly a good idea to get started but, you will only experience real success and deep meaning if you truly invest time and effort in reaching the goal. The more time, planning, and emotions you invest in this concept, the greater the results will be. Your comfort zone will be wider and more solid and you will know better what is not good for you and make decisions accordingly.

ENJOY will also not work if you rely too much on others. Like I said, there will always be skeptics. Don't let yourself be led astray. Develop confidence in your own talents and follow your own plan. The successes you will have as a result are worth so much more than any feedback you might expect from a "friend"—and then don't end up getting. Believe me, your world and those that belong in it will change.

There is a clear division—some will continue to believe that it is better to look for faults. Then there is you, who believes that people are inherently good and that it makes much more sense to invest in the capabilities, facts, and talents of each and every one of us. Be prepared, and then ask yourself, "What makes more sense for me? What price am I willing to pay?"

It is about your happiness, your health, and your future. Therefore, we must sometimes learn to let go of things we thought were a part of us. This book is not intended to replace any form of therapy. I want to emphasize this at this point as well. Those who have psychological problems should seek the help of loving hands who can understand them and help them professionally.

Summary

You have everything you need within you to become and be happy. You are unique, original beings with a very special task: to be yourself!

Stress and burnout prevention can only be solved on the individual, personal level. To be able to achieve this goal, your first obligation is to recognize what makes you unique, to understand who you are, and to truly appreciate and love yourself just the way you are. When you also understand what basic needs have to be met so you can be yourself, you have come a long way.

The next step will follow all by itself—because when you are proud of who you are and love yourself the way you are, you no longer feel the need to be somebody you are not. Comparisons will no longer be necessary; you are good enough. No, more than good enough. Unique— because no one has the same combination of talents you have. Therefore, it does not make any sense to compare yourself to anyone else.

What are the inherent values and talents you possess that motivate you to get out of bed in the morning, to start the day with gratitude, and fall into bed each night with a smile on your face, knowing that you did what you do best? That you've done a favor for yourself and those around you, and are glad to be able to get up again the next morning?

If you use your own talents and strengths in both your professional and private life as a basis for communicating with each individual, recognize and appreciate the uniqueness of every one, and recognize what you have and what you can give, the world will be a place in which we all have an opportunity to grow. When you reach that point, then stress and burnout will finally cease to spread fear and terror. Instead, stress will once again be seen as the lifesaver it was meant to be. Companies will be able to spend their money on further training their employees, instead of managing their stress.

ENJOY is a process for managing stress and burnout. But, it's also a plan you can use to live a life what is really YOUR life. It's a plan to develop yourself to become more self-aware, independent and bold to ask for the life you deserve.

It illustrates how I think and work—but it is only a part of the process. Unfortunately, it is not possible to cover the entire process as part of this book. I would be happy to talk to you about further details.

Please visit my website at www.strengths4you.com or send me an email to Nicole@strengths4you.com.

Start YOUR life. Make **ENJOY** a part of your life starting today!

ENJOY is my way to say thank you to life and to give back what I have been gifted!

Thank You

It is my mission, to make people smile, to make them happy. This is the message I got from God and what urged me to never give up. Many people along the way underestimated my persistence and mission. But even more people supported me on my way. And at this point I want to acknowledge them. I will try to name the most important ones—but please feel included even if you can't find your name.

First of all, I thank God for gifting me with the talents I have and for giving me the guidance to understand the power behind them. Thank you for connecting me with Clifton Strengths®, the language I needed to become your servant to help many people out there to become more of who they already are—by embracing their unique combination of talents to protect themselves from stress and burnout.

In the first place—thank you to my family. Thank you, for accepting every challenge with which I presented you. Especially while writing this book and even more in the last phase to finish this project. I don't have Achiever® high in my Clifton Strengths®. I love to start things but with this book I had to pull on my Belief® and Connectedness® to get it done. I just knew I had to do it. So thank you guys—for your patience and understanding. Lucas, Luis and Lena—I promise you will enjoy more of my kitchen skills again after this book has been published ☺. I love you so much.

Thank you Ute, it is because of you that I started to put my observations and pain in words—why can we not appreciate each other—and became a coach. I will always be grateful for that.

Thank you my dear friends Mirko, Ania, Katrin, Hans, Petra, Markus, Connie, Nicole, Helga, Helen, Diane and Robin for your unconditional love, You gifted me with the food for my soul and filled my bucket over and over again in the moments when I needed it most.

Thank you Helmut and Carmen—your love and positivity was always a shining star for me.

Thank you Dr. Donald O. Clifton for gifting this world with the best tool ever!

Thank you Mara Hoogerhuis and Jillian Anderson—for changing my life!

Thank you Adam Hickman and Jim Collison—your friendship and support was and is deeply appreciated.

Thank you MaryAnn Rivers—you have always been the kind of coach I wanted to become. You are a great role model and real friend.

Thank you to the team of Nicole Gebhardt, Crystal Yeagy and Maggie Petrovic, from Niche Pressworks. Without you guys this book couldn't be as strong as it is! You completed my mosaic with your brilliant knowledge and wisdom. Thank you so, so much.

And finally a thank you to my Mom. Because of you I became the woman I am today. For sure I challenged you a lot—I think I would have been a challenge for anyone. You gave your best—the foundation for me to become more of who I already was.

Notes - Inspirations

Kiefer. Lalouschek. (2009). Stressfood. Wien. Donauland.

Bell. Goldsmith. (2013).Managers as mentors. San Francisco. Berrett-Koehler Publishers.

Warren, Richard, 1954-. (2002). The purpose-driven life : what on earth am I here for? Grand Rapids, Mich. :Zondervan.

Huffington, A. (2016) . The sleep revolution. London. Ebury Publishing.

Unger. Kleinschmidt. (2011) . Bevor der Job krank macht. München. Kösel.

Heinemann. (2012) .Warum Burnout nicht vom Job kommt. Asslar. adeo.

Johnson,C. (2013). On target living. New Jersey. John Wiley & Sons, Inc.

Gloubermann,D. (2003) .The joy of burnout. Shanklin. Skyros.

Hanson,R. (2009). Buddha's brain.

Nuernberger,P. (1997). The quest for personal power. New York. The Berkley Pub. Group.

Burish. (1989). Das Burnout Syndrom. Berlin. Springer.

Stringer. (2016). The healthy workplace. New York. American Management Association.

Kaluza. (2004). Stressbewältigung. Berlin. Springer.

Mosetter. Cavelius,A. (2012). Die 4 Kräfte der Selbstheilung. Gräfe und Unzer.

Dr. Flemmer. (2011). Mood-Food-Glücksnahrung. Hannover. Schlütersche.

Dharma Singh Khalsa. (1997) .Brain Longevity. London. Century.

Michael Gershon. (2003). The second brain. New York, NY. Quill.

Karalus. Dr. Lindschinger. (2013). Iss dich schön, klug und sexy. München. riva.

About the Author

Born and raised in Germany, I started my journey as a coach because I wanted to change the world. It didn't feel right how people didn't appreciate and accept human uniqueness. I had a degree in Economics, but left the corporate world to change the world. And, it bothered me greatly that everyone was focused on fixing their own weaknesses instead of honoring the areas of excellence.

I added one coaching tool to the next—yet was still looking for something special to convince my clients why it makes so much more sense to look for the beauty in themselves, instead of fighting to be someone else. During this time, I connected the dots and became aware of how deeply connected our own happiness is to resilience of feeling stressed and experiencing a burnout.

In 2013, my journey brought me to the United States of America. Here is where I found what I was missing—the glue to connect all the pieces I had collected over the years. I found the language to explain the human uniqueness that I recognized was in each and every one of us – Clifton Strengths®.

I became a Gallup-Certified Clifton Strengths® Coach. Clifton Strengths® became the foundation of the work I was doing with corporate business as well as individuals. Strengths-based stress and burnout prevention. Understand who you are, create your unique comfort zone built from your unique combination of talents and align your life and your goals.

Honoring and protecting the human uniqueness is the best stress prevention ever. My ENJOY process is a simple way to do this! This is how I work with individuals and organizations. As a result, you will experience a new way to communicate. A new company culture will evolve. Let's get started.

ENJOY - Strengths Based Stress and Burnout Prevention.

Gallup Clifton Strengths® Coaching for individuals and organizations.

Gallup Q12® and Employee Engagement.

Visit my website www.strengths4you.com or send me an email at Nicole@strengths4you.com.

Special Offer

If this book and message has inspired you, we want to invite you to take the next step. This step would be to have an appointment with me to understand how you could benefit by implementing the ENJOY process in your life.

ENJOY for <u>You</u>

- 60-minute session with us.
- Review of your CliftonStrengths Top 5 Talent Theme report.
- Your goals and your values.
- Introduction to ENJOY.
- What are your challenges and how could ENJOY support you?
- Introduction to your ENJOY plan.
- Your next steps.
- Special offer during publishing of ENJOY US$ 99.00.

This session will provide you with a clear idea about how you can use the ENJOY process to achieve your goals and use your unique combination of talents on a daily base and how your combination of talents presents you with lots of opportunities to prevent stress and burnout. Let's get started.

Send us an email (**Nicole@strengths4you.com**) or visit our website **www.strengths4you.com**.

Special Offer

If this book and message has inspired you, we want to invite you to take the next step. This step would be to have an appointment with me to understand how your organization could benefit by implementing the ENJOY process and how you could create a new company culture.

ENJOY for
<u>Your Organization</u>

- 90-minute session with us.
- Review of your Clifton Strengths® top 5 talent theme report.
- Your challenges and pain points.
- Introduction to the ENJOY process.
- How do you address talent retention?
- How do you attract new talent?
- Introduction to the ENJOY plan for your organization.
- Your next steps.
- Special offer during publishing of ENJOY US$ 149.00.

This session will provide you with a clear idea about how you can use the ENJOY process to achieve your goals and improve the process within your organization. How can you implement strengths-based development in your organization? Where are your opportunities to create a solid and inspiring program to prevent stress and burnout in your organization?

Send us an email (**Nicole@strengths4you.com**) or visit our website **www.strengths4you.com**.